S0-FJW-848

MULTIPLE MINI INTERVIEW (MMI)

WINNING STRATEGIES FROM ADMISSIONS FACULTY

SAMIR P. DESAI MD
RAJANI KATTA MD

FROM THE AUTHORS OF THE SUCCESSFUL MATCH

PUBLISHED BY
MD2B
HOUSTON, TEXAS

www.MD2B.net

Multiple Mini Interview (MMI): Winning Strategies From Admissions Faculty is published by MD2B, PO Box 300988, Houston, TX 77230-0988.

www.MD2B.net
www.TheSuccessfulMatch.com

NOTICE: The authors and publisher disclaim any personal liability, either directly or indirectly, for advice or information presented within. The authors and publishers have used care and diligence in the preparation of this book. Every effort has been made to ensure the accuracy and completeness of information contained within this book. The reader should understand, however, that most of the book's subject matter is not rooted in scientific observation. The recommendations made within this book have come from the author's personal experiences and interactions with faculty, residents, and students over many years. There is considerable variability in the admissions process from one medical school to another. Therefore, the recommendations are not universally applicable. No responsibility is assumed for errors, inaccuracies, omissions, or any false or misleading implication that may arise due to the text.

© 2022 by Samir P. Desai and Rajani Katta

Contributing Author:
Dina Zamil BSc, author Chapter 14/ Case 6, Chapter 15/ Case 2, Chapter 16/ Case 2 and Chapter 20/ Case 2
Dina Zamil is a medical student at the Baylor College of Medicine.

Book Designer:
Veronica Perez Sanchez BSc, Public Health, is a graduate of Texas A&M University.

All rights reserved

No part of this publication may be reproduced, stored in a retrieval system, or transmitted, in any form or by any means, electronic, mechanical, photocopying, recording, or otherwise, without the prior written permission of the publisher.

Printed in the United States of America

ISBN #: 9781937978112

Dedication

To all of the front-line workers

Dedication

To all of the front-line workers

ABOUT THE AUTHORS

Samir P. Desai, M.D.

Dr. Samir Desai serves on the faculty of the Baylor College of Medicine in the Department of Medicine. He has educated premedical students, medical students, residents, and international medical graduates, work for which he has received numerous teaching awards. He is an author and editor, having written 21 books that together have sold over 250,000 copies worldwide.

He is the co-author of the *Medical School Interview: Winning Strategies from Admissions Faculty*, a highly acclaimed book that has helped thousands of applicants deliver a compelling and powerful interview performance. He has spoken about interview success at universities across the country and leads the medical school interview workshop at Rice University.

His book *Success in Medical School: Insider Advice for the Preclinical Years* provides preclinical students with detailed knowledge and guidance to excel in medical school. To help students lower the cost of attending medical school and position themselves for residency match success, he wrote the book *Medical School Scholarships, Grants, & Awards*.

He is also the co-author of *Success on the Wards: 250 Rules for Clerkship Success*. This book has helped students make the difficult transition from the preclinical to clinical years of medical school. *Success on the Wards* is a required or recommended resource at many U.S. medical schools.

He is also the co-creator of Medical School Interviewing 101, the course that helps premed students quickly and confidently prepare for their medical school interviews, using before-and-after videos and a step-by-step approach.

As a faculty member, he has served on the medical school admissions and residency selection committees. His commitment to helping premedical and medical students reach their professional goals led him to develop the website TheSuccessfulMatch.com. The website's mission is to provide medical school and residency applicants with a better understanding of the selection process. Applicants interested in partnering with Dr. Desai to elevate their interview performance can learn more about his medical school mock interview service at TheSuccessfulMatch.com.

After completing his residency training in Internal Medicine at Northwestern University in Chicago, Dr. Desai had the opportunity to serve as chief medical resident. He received his M.D. degree from Wayne State University School of Medicine in Detroit, Michigan, graduating first in his class.

He now resides in Houston, TX with his wife (and co-author) Dr. Rajani Katta and their two children.

Rajani Katta, M.D.

Dr. Rajani Katta is an award-winning educator who is deeply passionate about patient, medical student, and physician education.

She served as Professor of Dermatology at the Baylor College of Medicine for over 17 years, and founded the Baylor College of Medicine Contact Dermatitis Clinic. In 2015 she left to establish her own practice dedicated to allergic contact dermatitis.

She has authored over 90 scientific articles and chapters, and has lectured extensively both nationally and locally on dermatology and contact dermatitis to students, residents, and physicians. On a national level, she has worked closely to advance the mission of the American Contact Dermatitis Society, serving on the Board of Directors.

She has been deeply involved in medical student education. She served as Course Director for Dermatology for 15 years, and previously served as Clerkship Director of Dermatology.

She is also the co-creator of Medical School Interviewing 101, the course that uses before-and-after videos and a step-by-step approach to help applicants go from good to great to unforgettable. Having advised many students over the years regarding the dermatology match process, she was determined to become an expert in this area. She co-authored *The Successful Match: 200 Rules to Succeed in the Residency Match*. The book quickly became the best-selling title in this field. It has been recommended as Suggested Reading in the AAMC Careers in Medicine Student Guide and identified as a high-value resource by the AAMC Group on Student Affairs.

She has authored a total of 7 books. One of these books, *Success on the Wards: 250 Rules for Clerkship Success*, has helped thousands of medical students make the difficult transition from the preclinical to clinical years of medical school. *Success on the Wards* is a required or recommended resource at numerous US medical schools.

She has a strong interest in preventive dermatology and has written frequently on the link between diet and dermatology. She maintains a blog at KattaMD.com, with the goal of helping foster better dietary choices by emphasizing the effects of diet on the skin. She has been interviewed frequently on this topic, and has been featured in or quoted by all of the major news networks and many media outlets, including CNN, the New York Times, Oprah magazine, Today.com, and many others.

After graduating with honors from Baylor College of Medicine and completing her internship in Internal Medicine, she completed her dermatology residency at the Northwestern University School of Medicine.

She and her husband Dr. Samir Desai (her co-author) have two children and one frog and reside in Houston, Texas. They enjoy hiking, and love to hear about great hikes.

How Else Can We Help You Get Into Med School?

Visit us at TheSuccessfulMatch.com for more MMI examples and expert interview techniques.

For more resources to help you prepare for traditional and behavioral interview questions please see our course

Medical School Interviewing 101

The course uses before-and-after videos and our expert step-by-step approach to help you quickly and confidently prepare for your traditional medical school interview.

For more information visit us at
TheInterviewCourse.com

Don't forget about our book for the traditional medical school interview:

The Medical School Interview: Winning Strategies from Admissions Faculty

CONTENTS

TABLE OF CONTENTS: SCENARIOS AND QUESTIONS

TABLE OF CONTENTS: SCENARIOS AND QUESTIONS

TABLE OF CONTENTS: SCENARIOS AND QUESTIONS

Chapter 1

Introduction

"Finally!" The patient, visibly frustrated, continued loudly with his complaint. "I'm in so much pain. That last nurse did nothing for me. I kept calling for her, and it took an eternity for her to come. That went on all night long. I couldn't sleep. I couldn't rest. It's like she was watching TV or something. I hope you can do better."

This is the type of exchange that could occur in any hospital. However, this particular encounter took place, not in a hospital, but during a medical school interview.

Playing the role of nurse was Sarah, a 25-year-old applicant who had desperately wanted to become a physician ever since childhood. Her chances of success hinged on her ability to interact effectively with an actor playing the role of an angry patient.

Early in college, Sarah had suffered from a variety of symptoms that left her weak and tired. Multiple visits to specialist after specialist failed to yield a diagnosis, and Sarah's grades suffered. One year later, with diagnosis finally in hand, she was appropriately treated and made a full recovery. By that time, however, the damage had been done and her GPA had plummeted.

Determined to reach her professional dreams, Sarah persisted and excelled in her remaining courses. Hopeful that medical schools would understand her situation, she applied as a college senior. She failed to receive even a single interview. After meeting with an advisor, it was clear that her biggest obstacle was a low GPA.

Following graduation, she enrolled in a two-year post-baccalaureate program. Several months into this new program, she applied again to medical school. Sadly, the outcome was the same. Although initially shaken, she persevered and maintained a 4.0 GPA.

In the fall of her second year as a post-baccalaureate student, she opened an email. "Thank you for applying to…After careful review of your application materials, our admissions committee would like to invite you for an interview…" It was her third attempt, and she was elated to see that her hard work and determination had finally paid dividends. Now all that remained between her and a seat in medical school was the admissions interview.

At this particular school, a relatively new and innovative interview technique, known as the multiple mini interview (MMI), was in place. To understand why, it helps to trace the origins of the MMI. In 2001, on the west end of Lake Ontario, in an area known as the Golden Horseshoe, a small group of medical school educators at the Michael G. DeGroote School of Medicine at McMaster University initiated an interesting pilot project. Eighteen graduate students were recruited to act as "medical school candidates." These students were asked to participate in a series of brief interviews. Each interview station was designed to measure a certain non-cognitive quality or skill deemed important in future doctors. Interviewees interacted with a different interviewer or rater at each station.

Promising results led to a larger, more robust study in 2002, this time with real medical school candidates. As the data was analyzed, it became clear that the educators were on to something big. The new interview technique showed high overall test reliability.[1] Subsequent research demonstrated that it was superior to the traditional interview as a predictor of medical school clinical performance.[2]

Just two years later, in 2004, McMaster University introduced the MMI to the world of medical school admissions. Since then, the MMI has been adopted by numerous medical schools. Its reach has expanded beyond medical schools to include veterinary, dentistry, and pharmacy schools. In 2008, the University of Cincinnati College of Medicine became the first medical school in the United States to adopt this new interview technique. Since then, interest in MMI has exploded among allopathic and osteopathic medical schools. At the time of this book's writing, over 50 U.S. medical schools utilized the MMI in the admissions process.

For medical school applicants, the MMI's arrival represented a major change in the medical school admissions process. Change, especially in the high stakes world of admissions, often causes great anxiety for students, parents, and advisors, and the MMI was no exception. For years, medical schools had utilized the traditional interview format, a one-on-one or panel-based interview experience where applicants answered questions, such as "Tell me about yourself" and "Why do you want to be a doctor?"

Many students spent months preparing for the traditional interview, and there was a plethora of books available to help guide preparation. There were also numerous advisors skilled in mock interviewing. With enough practice and the right guidance, students could feel confident in their interview skills.

With the arrival of the MMI, everything changed. To maintain validity and objectivity, medical schools began requiring interviewees to sign forms preventing release of MMI information to others. On discussion forums, medical students who had taken part in MMIs were relegated to delivering generic advice such as "Be yourself and try to enjoy it."

Advisors and applicants turned to the Internet for more specific information. At the websites of those schools utilizing the MMI format, little could be found beyond basic information about its structure and the reasons why schools chose to adopt the new technique. "The strongest advice is to understand the basic structure, time limit, and number of stations," wrote one school in the South.[3] "It is not recommended that you try to prepare for specific MMI questions," wrote another school.[4]

Sarah faced these challenges when she prepared for the MMI. With a dearth of specific information to guide her preparation, she felt understandably nervous on her interview day.

How did Sarah handle the opening scenario?

Prior to entering the room with the actor playing the angry patient, Sarah was given the following information:

During shift change, your nurse colleague informs you of a "problem patient" that you will be taking care of. She reports being "harassed" all night long by repeated requests for more pain medication. "I followed the doctor's orders, and there was no extra pain medication I could give." As the night progressed, their encounters became increasingly tense and hostile. "I gave him pain medication about an hour ago. He's not due for more for another two hours. Good luck with this one," she says. "You're going to really need it." Enter the room as the patient's new nurse.

Patient: Finally. I'm in so much pain. That last nurse did nothing for me. I kept calling for her, and it took an eternity for her to come. That went on all night long. I couldn't sleep. I couldn't rest. It's like she was watching TV or something. I hope you can do better.

Nurse Sarah: Well, I can promise you that she wasn't watching TV. What can I help you with?

Patient: Haven't you heard anything that I've said? I need some pain medication. How about getting me some? The other nurse told me to try some breathing exercises. Can you believe that? We're talking about real pain here. Eleven out of ten, do you hear me?

Nurse Sarah: I'm sure it's eleven out of ten. Now, we've already...

Patient: I don't like your condescending tone.

Nurse Sarah: I wasn't being condescending. What I was trying to say when you interrupted me was that you've already been given pain medication. You're not due for another dose for another two hours.

Patient: Are you kidding me? I'm trying to tell you that I'm in pain. And you're telling me that I have to wait for two hours. Do you know where the doctor is? Why don't you call him? You and that other nurse – I don't get it. Why did you go into nursing? You're supposed to help people.

Nurse Sarah: The pain medication that's been ordered has been given to you. I really think you should calm down. Maybe if you do, your pain would be more tolerable.

Patient: How dare you tell me to calm down? I demand to talk to your supervisor. I'm going to tell her that you're refusing to give me pain medication.

Nurse Sarah: I've already told you. There's no medication that anyone's holding. You've gotten what's written for.

Patient: Just call the doctor. And bring the nurse supervisor in too.

Analyzing Sarah's answer

Sarah left the encounter frustrated. What went wrong? How could she have avoided this outcome? The angry patient or person scenario is frequently part of the MMI circuit. As you read through Sarah's dialogue with the patient, were you able to identify the factors that led to this unsuccessful encounter? I've listed and described these in the following box.

It was obvious that the patient was upset but Sarah **did not acknowledge** the patient's emotions or feelings. "You seem very upset" would have been one way for Sarah to do so.

Sarah never invited the patient to **share his story** and fully vent. It was clear that the patient had much on his mind. Sarah needed to make the patient feel that he was being heard.

Sarah **failed to show sympathy** or regret for the patient's situation. "I'm really sorry you had to go through all this" would have been effective.

Sarah **lost her composure**. At one point, the patient commented on her condescending tone. At another point, Sarah asked the patient to "calm down." Setting limits when someone is angry is seldom effective. In such situations, it's important to keep your cool.

Sarah **never explored any other solutions**. A particularly effective technique is to ask the patient for his thoughts on possible solutions. "Do you have some suggestions on ways to solve the problem?" Through this process, Sarah may have been able to **find an acceptable solution**. "Here's what I suggest…"

The angry patient is a common scenario in the MMI because it's such a common scenario in medicine. Patients, when faced with the stress of illness, sometimes act in uncharacteristic ways. They may lash out at their doctors and nurses for many reasons. Being sick enough to be hospitalized is frightening for most people. Patients commonly feel afraid, confused, and powerless. They feel that they have no control over what's happening to them. Physical factors, such as acute or chronic pain, may also play a role. Dealing with bad news that impacts prognosis, dealing with the risk of a disability, and the realities of living with a life-threatening illness: all of these are obviously severe stressors.

Sometimes the healthcare system itself can be the cause, as in long waiting times for a test, or an intrusive procedure, or denied insurance claims. At other times, the patient-physician relationship will cause a patient to lash out, such as when a physician is perceived as arrogant or disrespectful. Understand that there may be a number of factors at play when a patient lashes out at you, and that, in most cases, you shouldn't take it personally.

Sarah clearly didn't perform well during this scenario. Fortunately for Sarah, this wasn't a real admissions interview. This was a mock interview experience in which I played the role of patient. After I analyzed her performance, Sarah was able to better understand where things went wrong. She was then able to implement several strategies to effectively handle this type of situation, as you'll see in the following encounter.

You are the nurse manager on a busy hospital floor. One of your nurses is upset after a difficult patient encounter. The patient was in considerable pain but the nurse was unable to give him anything because the next dose of pain medication was not scheduled for another several hours. As she tried to explain the situation, the patient became quite angry and questioned the nurse's dedication to her profession. Hurt by this, the nurse lost control of her emotions, and the situation escalated, with the patient requesting to speak with the nurse manager. The patient is now waiting for you in the room. Enter the room.

Nurse Manager Sarah:	Hello Mr. Smith. I'm the nurse manager on the floor. I understand you wanted to speak with me. How are you feeling?
Patient:	Terrible. I'm in a lot of pain and no one seems to care.
Nurse Manager Sarah:	Can you tell me what happened?
Patient:	I just want some medication to help me with this pain. It's now so bad – nine out of ten. I've just been sitting here hoping and waiting for medication. The nurse told me that if I calmed down, that I might feel better. Can you believe that? I need some pills or even a shot. I need something. I'm really hurting.
Nurse Manager Sarah:	So let me see if I've understood the situation. You're in a lot of pain, and you don't feel like the current pain medication is providing you with enough relief.
Patient:	Yes, that's what I'm saying. I need something stronger than what I'm getting. I told the nurse this, and she kept telling me to calm down. I asked her to help me, and she kept telling me that it wasn't time for the next dose. I asked her to call the doctor, and she didn't look too happy about that.
Nurse Manager Sarah:	I'm sorry that you're in so much pain. It sounds like you would find it helpful if I reached out to your doctor. That's something I can do. I'll call and let him know that your pain medication is not keeping the pain under control. Perhaps he can make an adjustment to the medication or stop by and take a look at you.
Patient:	I would love that. I don't know why it's so hard to find the doctor.

Nurse Manager Sarah:	Let me go and call the doctor. Let's see if we can come up with a plan to address this. How does that sound to you?
Patient:	That sounds wonderful.
Nurse Manager Sarah:	Before I take care of that, I wanted to see what else I can do for you. I know you're uncomfortable, and I apologize for that. Is there anything else I can do to help you? Are you cold? Do you need a blanket? How about a snack?
Patient:	Would you mind turning the TV on for me?

In the following pages, you'll learn how to create this type of response.

A response that confirms that you have the qualities that this medical school seeks. The type of response that confirms to the interviewer that you are the perfect fit for their medical school.

In the next 350+ pages, we'll review, in depth, the multiple mini interview. You'll learn how critical the interview is in the admissions process. The Association of American Medical Colleges (AAMC) evaluated the importance of 12 variables on admissions decisions.[5] Of these, the MCAT score was rated sixth. Cumulative science and math GPA was rated third. What was the most important variable?

The most important factor in admissions decisions was, in fact, the interview.

You'll learn why the MMI is so important to admissions officers. It's widely recognized that the best physicians have more than just great scores and grades. The most effective physicians display a number of non-academic attributes. These traits are difficult to evaluate, and admissions officers rely on the MMI to help assess these traits. "Our school intends to graduate physicians who can communicate with patients and work in a team," writes Dr. Cynda Johnson, Dean of the Virginia Tech Carilion School of Medicine. "So if people do poorly on the MMI, they will not be offered positions in our class."[6]

How can you tell which qualities will be measured during your MMI? Unless you're privy to inside information at that school, you can't know for sure. However, every school will create its MMI to assess for those qualities or skills that it has deemed important in its future students. In Chapter 3, we'll show you how to determine those qualities and skills.

We also review, in detail, other important aspects of the MMI. You'll understand who the raters (interviewers) are, how they'll interact with you, and what they're looking for. In Chapter 5, you'll also learn about their pet peeves, as well as the behaviors and attitudes that would lead them to flag you as an unsuitable candidate. Will your interviewers challenge you? They absolutely will, and I'll show you how to respond to these probing questions in a compelling manner. What else do you need to be concerned about? In one study, researchers described the concerns raised by interviewers who had been tasked with asking applicants certain interview questions. A major concern involved "assessor fatigue." What is it, and how could it affect your performance?[7]

You'll also hear from interviewees. In one study, 10% of participants rated the MMI as worse than the traditional interview.[7] What were the problem areas cited by interviewees? What caused them the most difficulty? How can you avoid their mistakes?

"There are no right or wrong answers," writes one Midwestern U.S. medical school.[8] Is that true? Are there really no right or wrong answers? As reassuring as this sounds, there are clearly wrong answers. In Chapter 7, we'll present the types of answers that can remove an applicant from consideration. You'll see how such answers can easily surface in the high stakes setting of the MMI. You'll learn how to avoid these responses, and deliver answers that yield high interview scores.

We break down the process of developing and delivering powerful answers to MMI questions in chapters 8 – 12. You'll then be able to utilize these strategies with our example questions. This will help provide the practice needed to elevate your performance. With each question, task, or scenario, we provide a sample answer with a thorough explanation of what makes the response so effective.

The recommendations in this book are based on multiple sources. Throughout the book, you'll see quotes from many different admissions officers. Although the MMI is a relatively new interview technique, there's been a substantial body of research on the topic. We've included the results of these research studies, which have shaped and guided our recommendations. Lastly, the recommendations are based on extensive discussions with applicants as well as admissions faculty. Dr. Desai served on the admissions committee at the Baylor College of Medicine for over 10 years, and has interacted with admissions officials at numerous medical schools. Dr. Katta served on the residency selection committee for over 15 years. We now provide interview preparation services, and have worked with numerous medical school applicants. (To see where our students have been accepted, please see our website www.TheSuccessfulMatch.com. Our student acceptances cover almost every state in the United States.) In this book, as in our previous books, we've applied a combination of evidence-based advice and insider knowledge.

We've seen where students have excelled in interviews, and we've seen where they've failed. In the next 400+ pages, you'll learn how to apply these lessons to your own interview preparation. It's taken years of intense work for you to reach this point, and receiving an invitation to interview is a strong vote of confidence from the medical school. In the following pages, you'll learn how to make the most of this opportunity in order to reach your goal: medical school.

References

[1]Eva K, Reiter H, Rosenfeld J, Norman G. An admissions OSCE: the multiple mini-interview. *Med Educ* 2004; 38: 314-26.
[2]Reiter H, Eva K, Rosenfeld J, Norman G. Multiple mini-interview predicts for clinical clerkship performance, National Licensure Examination Performance. *Med Educ* 2007; 41(4): 378-84.
[3]Duke University School of Medicine. Available at: http://dukemed.duke.edu/modules/ooa_applicant/print.php?id=9. Accessed May 12, 2015.
[4]University of Nevada School of Medicine. Available at: http://medicine.nevada.edu/asa/admissions/applicants/selection-factors/applicant-interviews. Accessed May 12, 2015.
[5]Dunleavy D, Sondheimer H, Bletzinger R, Castillo-Page L. Medical school admissions: more than grades and test scores. *AIB* 2011: 11 (6).
[6]New York Times. Available at: http://www.nytimes.com/2011/07/11/health/policy/11docs.html?_r=0. Accessed May 3, 2015.
[7]McAndrew R, Ellis J. An evaluation of the multiple mini-interview as a selection tool for dental students. *Br Dent J* 2012; 212 (7): 331-5.
[8]Michigan State University College of Human Medicine. Available at: http://mdadmissions.msu.edu/applicants/mmi_faq.php. Accessed May 4, 2015.

Chapter 2

The MMI and its Importance in the Admissions Process

Rule # 1   **The medical school interview is a critical factor in the medical school admissions process.**

When applying to medical school, the admissions interview is a critical factor. In fact, at some schools it's the most important factor. In one survey of medical schools, over 60% of surveyed schools reported that the admissions interview was the most important factor in the selection process.[1]

One survey provides further data. The Association of American Medical Colleges (AAMC) published a survey that evaluated the importance of 12 variables on admissions decisions. These variables included total MCAT scores, science and math GPA, and the interview. Many students are surprised by the results.

Of the 12 variables, total MCAT score was rated sixth in importance. Cumulative science and math GPA was rated third.[2]

What was the most important factor? The most important factor in admissions decisions was in fact the interview. The interview received a mean importance rating of 4.5 (scale of 1 [not important] to 5 [extremely important]).

Did you know…

Data published by the AAMC (Association of American Medical Colleges) indicates that even high-achieving applicants are often denied medical school admission. For applicants with both a GPA greater than 3.79 and an MCAT score of 514 and higher, almost 20% failed to gain admission to medical school.

Why is the interview considered so important, especially in relation to factors such as MCAT scores and science GPAs? "Medical educators agree that success in medical school requires more than academic competence," wrote the authors. "It also requires integrity, altruism, self-management, interpersonal and teamwork skills, among other characteristics."[2] Medical school faculty have long known that while academic variables such as scores and grades may predict preclinical performance, they're not as helpful in predicting which students will become good physicians. Studies have shown that scores and grades don't have as much predictive power, with respect to clinical performance, as do other factors.[3]

What does predict clinical performance? In one study, interview ratings of nonacademic attributes correlated strongly with subjective evaluations of clinical performance in required clerkships. These nonacademic attributes included interpersonal skills, maturity, and motivation/interest in medicine.[4]

Given these findings, med schools can't rely solely on objective data such as scores and grades. Noncognitive skills have significant value in predicting clinical performance, and since schools are limited as to how they can assess such skills, the interview takes on greater importance.

Importance of the Admissions Interview Based On Review of Medical School Websites	
Medical School	**Website Comments**
Vanderbilt University	Interviews are an important part of the application process because it provides the admissions committee with the opportunity to evaluate an applicant's interpersonal skills and intangible qualities that cannot be evaluated through MCAT scores, GPA, or other parts of the application.[5]
University of Connecticut	An important part of the admissions committee's final selections, the interview provides an opportunity to meet the applicant and to gather additional personal and supplemental data for the committee to evaluate the applicant…Interviews provide the admissions committee with personal impressions and insights on the applicant by evaluating, and putting in perspective, all aspects of the applicant's background, experiences coursework, motivations, and values.[6]
UCLA	The interview is an important and integral part of the selection process. It gives the Admissions Committee an opportunity to learn more about the candidate and their ability to be part of the entering class.[7]
Penn State University	The interview is an essential component of the selection process. It provides vital information about the applicant that is impossible to obtain by any other means. Faculty interviews with critical evaluations are the only method within the admissions process for the assessment of the important nonacademic attributes of applicants. The Selection Committee places great importance on these evaluations in making decisions on admission.[8]
LSU Shreveport	High grades and/or MCAT scores alone are never enough. For those interviewed, impressions from the personal interview are exceedingly important.[9]

Rule # 2   Understand why some medical schools have
                                replaced the traditional interview with the MMI

As a faculty member who has served on the medical school admissions
and residency selection committees at several U.S. medical schools, I
have been privy to some interesting discussions about applicants. Here
is an example of what you may hear in an admissions committee meeting
at med schools utilizing a traditional interview format:

Did you know…

In the United States, the most common interview format is the traditional one-on-one
interview. With this format, the interviewer will typically ask questions about your
education, activities, and goals. Examples include:

- Tell me about yourself.
- What are your strengths?
- Why are you interested in our medical school?

Interviewer # 1: I was really looking forward to meeting Lisa. Her
application indicated that she was someone who was really committed to
caring for the underserved. Early in her college career, she had become
involved in the local area free health clinic. Her personal statement
indicates that this experience was very meaningful to her, and it certainly
seems that she was highly regarded by the clinic staff. In her junior year,
she was given the title of Patient Assistance Representative. In this
position, she had extensive patient contact, and was the point person for
working with pharmaceutical companies to obtain medication free or at
reduced cost for the clinic's patients.

Needless to say, I wanted to learn more about all of this, but when I asked
her questions about her involvement, I was surprised by the superficiality
of her responses. I was really looking for depth in her answers, and I
couldn't find it no matter how hard I tried. Maybe it was because I was
her first interviewer, but I tried to get her to relax. She did seem nervous
at the beginning but I would say that her answers continued to be brief
and superficial throughout most of the interview. That's why I gave her
the score that I did.

Interviewer # 2: We did talk about her work in the free clinic, and I got
the sense that she found the entire experience very rewarding. I didn't
have any trouble talking to her, and found her very easy to talk to, really
quite engaging. It turns out that we went to the same college, so we had

a nice discussion about the campus, what she likes to do, and so on. I have to say that I was quite impressed with her enthusiasm and her maturity. I think that her life experiences would really add to the diversity of our class. I would love to see her here.

Interviewer # 1 was clearly excited to meet Lisa but was not impressed with her interview performance. She was particularly disappointed because Lisa's answers were brief and lacking in depth. Interviewer # 2 had a very different impression. He was struck by her enthusiasm, and felt that it was easy to connect with her.

As an admissions committee member, I would often listen to these discussions, and wonder if my colleagues had interviewed the same applicant. Why would two interviewers have such different opinions of the same applicant?

Studies of the traditional interview have found that interview ratings are significantly influenced by the biases, expectations, and perspectives of the individual interviewers.[10-12] While variance in interview ratings is multifactorial, research has shown that interviewer variability is a major factor, accounting for 56% of the variance in interview scores.[13] Limitations of the traditional interview are presented in the following box.

Limitations of the Traditional Interview

- Interviewer may be easily influenced by an early answer (positively or negatively)

- Interviewer brings a variety of biases into the encounter (conscious or unconscious)

- Scoring of interviewees varies from interviewer to interviewer, leading to inconsistency

- Considerable variability between interviewers

- Difficulty measuring non-cognitive qualities important in future physicians

---

The limitations of the traditional interview led researchers at McMaster University in Hamilton, Ontario to develop a new interview technique called the Multiple Mini-Interview (MMI).[14]

Admissions Officers Speak...

"Our school intends to graduate physicians who can communicate with patients and work in a team. So if people do poorly on the MMI, they will not be offered positions in our class."[15]

Dr. Cynda AnnJohnson, Dean of the Virginia Tech Carilion School of Medicine

----

"Approximately 12% of the hundreds of candidates interviewed each year at WesternU/COMP receive a 'Do not recommend' rating after their MMI performance."[16]

Western University of Health Sciences College of Osteopathic Medicine of the Pacific (in an interview with The DO)

"My bias is toward thoughtful, caring physicians who connect with the patient. We want leaders, but those with interpersonal skills and empathy. I do not want to graduate a medical student from our school who wouldn't be comfortable taking care of a patient."[17]

Dr. Charles Prober, Senior Associate Dean for Medical Education at the Stanford University School of Medicine

----

"MMI is an important tool to help the Admissions Committee gather information about the important characteristics physicians need to work effectively with patients and members of the health care team."[18]

University of Nevada School of Medicine

"The MMI and the holistic admissions model aren't just about which applicants have the best grades and MCAT scores, but which ones will make the best doctors."[19]

Dr. Nathan Smith, Assistant Dean for Admissions at University of Alabama at Birmingham School of Medicine

Rule # 3   **Understand how the MMI overcomes the limitations of the traditional interview.**

"We were really dissatisfied with the process for admitting students to medical school," said Jack Rosenfeld, Professor Emeritus of Pathology and Molecular Medicine and Co-Creator of the MMI, in an interview with The Globe and Mail. "There were students that got in and maybe shouldn't have."[20]

Researchers were also driven to develop this new interview approach to ensure that desirable candidates were not removed from consideration because of the limitations of the traditional interview. "With the traditional interview process, a terrific student could have a bad interview. With the MMI, a single bad review can be neutralized by the reviews by multiple other raters," said Dr. Mariann Manno, Interim Associate Dean for Admission at the University of Massachusetts Medical School.[21]

The MMI method uses a structured and consistent approach with multiple raters. It has been shown to be reliable and more predictive of future performance in medical school, especially during clinical clerkships. In a study performed by researchers at McMaster University, MMI scores correlated well with clerkship and Objective Structured Clinical Examination (OSCE) evaluations.[22]

Advantages of MMI Over the Traditional Interview

- The MMI usually has 8 to 10 stations. At each station, there will be a different interviewer (rater). Therefore, you will be exposed to far more interviewers than you would during the typical traditional interview. These interactions will yield more data, and allow for a more accurate rating.

- Every applicant encounters the same questions, scenarios, and tasks at these stations. In other words, the MMI is standardized.

- Interviewers will not have access to the GPA and MCAT score. By blinding interviewers to the academic record, the MMI allows for a more objective evaluation of the traits and behaviors the school has deemed important in their future doctors.

Established in 2002, use of the MMI in U.S. medical schools has grown rapidly.

Did you know...

In 2021-2022, over 50 allopathic and osteopathic U.S. medical schools have reported that they will be using the MMI approach, either alone or in combination with the traditional interview.

A number of research studies have supported the utility of the MMI, and its use in the admissions process is likely to only increase in the future.

In one systematic review, MMIs used in the selection process at undergraduate health programs appear to have "reasonable feasibility, acceptability, validity, and reliability" [23] Overall, the MMI was felt to represent a non-biased selection tool on the basis of age, gender, and socioeconomic status. However, concerns remain about its use in those with low English proficiency, or for applicants of certain ethnic and social backgrounds, representing areas important for further research.

Some schools have extensively documented their implementation of the MMI format. For example, the University of North Carolina first convened 15 focus groups with students, educators, administrators, clinicians, and nursing teams. Each focus group was asked about the qualities that they thought the university should be looking for in medical students. Themes were identified and then iterated, resulting in a focus on seven skills. The university also consulted with other medical schools and programs, and sought input from faculty in the schools of Education and Business. Then, six stations were developed and pilot tested with medical students. [24]

In 2020, schools were able to adapt the MMI to a virtual format. Several schools have documented their successful implementation of a virtual MMI.[25,26] Although these involved a high level of organization and required significant support staff, the pivot to a virtual format was deemed successful. The University of Houston College of Medicine received preliminary accreditation in February 2020 and has described in detail its initiation of the virtual MMI. This involved a total of 7 MMI stations and made use of Zoom breakout rooms.[27]

More information on virtual MMIs, with recommendations on how to excel, are found in Chapter 4 The MMI Format.

U.S. Medical Schools Reporting Use of the MMI

*for the most up-to-date listing, please see AAMC resource Medical School Admission Requirements™ (MSAR®) Report for Applicants and Advisors: Interview Procedures

Alabama

University of Alabama Birmingham School of Medicine

Arizona

A.T. Still University School of Osteopathic Medicine in Arizona
University of Arizona College of Medicine-Phoenix
University of Arizona College of Medicine-Tucson

California

California Northstate University College of Medicine
Kaiser-Permanente School of Medicine
Stanford University School of Medicine
UC Davis School of Medicine
UC Riverside School of Medicine
UC San Diego School of Medicine
UCLA David Geffen School of Medicine
Western University of Health Sciences College of Osteopathic Medicine of the Pacific

Florida

Florida Atlantic University Charles E. Schmidt College of Medicine
Nova Southeastern University Dr. Kiran C. Patel College of Osteopathic Medicine

Georgia

Medical College of Georgia at Augusta University

Illinois

Chicago Medical School at Rosalind Franklin University of Medicine and Science
University of Illinois-Chicago College of Medicine

Indiana

Marian University College of Osteopathic Medicine

Massachusetts

University of Massachusetts Medical School

Michigan

Central Michigan University School of Medicine
Michigan State University College of Human Medicine
University of Michigan Medical School
Wayne State University School of Medicine

Minnesota

University of Minnesota School of Medicine (Twin Cities)

Mississippi

University of Mississippi Medical School

Missouri

University of Missouri-Kansas City School of Medicine

Nevada

University of Nevada School of Medicine

New Jersey

Cooper Medical School of Rowan University
UMDNJ-Robert Wood Johnson Medical School

New York

Albany Medical College
New York Medical College
New York University Grossman School of Medicine
New York University Long Island School of Medicine
SUNY Upstate Medical University
Zucker School of Medicine at Hofstra-Northwell

North Carolina

Duke University School of Medicine
University of North Carolina School of Medicine
Wake Forest University School of Medicine

Ohio

University of Cincinnati College of Medicine
University of Toledo College of Medicine

Oregon

Oregon Health & Science University

Texas

Dell Medical School at University of Texas Austin
Texas Christian University and UNT HSC School of Medicine
University of Houston College of Medicine
Texas College of Osteopathic Medicine
University of the Incarnate Word School of Osteopathic Medicine

Utah

University of Utah School of Medicine

Vermont

University of Vermont College of Medicine

Virginia

Virginia Commonwealth University School of Medicine
Virginia Tech Carilion School of Medicine

Washington

Pacific Northwest University of Health Sciences College of Osteopathic Medicine

Puerto Rico

San Juan Bautista School of Medicine
Universidad Central del Caribe School of Medicine

Canadian Medical Schools Utilizing MMI

Alberta

University of Alberta Faculty of Medicine and Dentistry
University of Calgary Faculty of Medicine

British Columbia

University of British Columbia Faculty of Medicine

Manitoba

University of Manitoba Faculty of Medicine

Newfoundland

Memorial University of Newfoundland Faculty of Medicine

Nova Scotia

Dalhousie University Faculty of Medicine

Ontario

McMaster University Michael G. DeGroote School of Medicine
Northern Ontario School of Medicine
Queen's University Faculty of Health Sciences

Quebec

Laval University Faculty of Medicine
McGill University Faculty of Medicine
University of Montreal Faculty of Medicine
University of Sherbrooke Faculty of Medicine

Saskatchewan

University of Saskatchewan College of Medicine

References

[1]Puryear J, Lewis L. Description of the interview process in selecting students for admission to U.S. medical schools. *J Med Educ* 1981; 56 (11): 881-85.

[2]Dunleavy D, Sondheimer H, Bletzinger R, Castillo-Page L. Medical school admissions: more than grades and test scores. *AIB* 2011: 11 (6).

[3]Mitchell K. Traditional predictors of performance in medical school. Paper presented at the annual meeting of the American Educational Research Association, San Francisco, California, March 1989.

[4]Meredith K, Dunlap M, Baker H. Subjective and objective admissions factors as predictors of clinical clerkship performance. *J Med Educ* 1982; 57: 743-51.

[5]Vanderbilt University School of Medicine. Available at: https://medschool.vanderbilt.edu/admissions/campus-interview. Accessed February 22, 2013.

[6]University of Connecticut School of Medicine. Available at: http://medicine.uchc.edu/prospective/apply/index.html. Accessed February 22, 2013.

[7]UCLA David Geffen School of Medicine. Available at: http://ww.medstudentucla.edu/offices/admiss/interv.cfm. Accessed February 22, 2013.

[8]Penn State University College of Medicine. Available at: http://www2.med.psu.edu/mdadmissions/interview-process/. Accessed February 21, 2013.

[9]LSU – Shreveport School of Medicine. Available at: http://www.lsuhscshreveport.edu/Admissions/ReApplicants.aspx#personal. Accessed February 22, 2013.

[10]Edwards J, Johnson E, Molidor J. The interview in the admission process. *Acad Med* 1990; 65: 167–75.

[11]Elam C, Andrykowksi M. Admission interview ratings: relationship to applicant academic and demographic variables and interviewer characteristics. *Acad Med* (Suppl) 1991; 66: 13–15.

[12]Elam CL, Johnson MM. An analysis of admission committee voting patterns. *Acad Med* (Suppl) 1997; 69: 72–755.

[13]Harasym P, Woloschuk W, Mandin H, Brundin-Mather R. Reliability and validity of interviewers' judgements of medical school candidates. *Acad Med* (Suppl) 1996; 71: 40–42.

[14]Eva K, Rosenfeld J, Reiter H, Norman G. An admissions OSCE: the multiple mini-interview. *Med Educ* 2004; 38 (3): 314-26.

[15]New York Times. Available at: http://www.nytimes.com/2011/07/11/health/policy/11docs.html?_r=0. Accessed May 3, 2015.

[16]The DO. Available at: http://thedo.osteopathic.org/2014/09/multple-mini-interviews-gains-traction-schools/. Accessed May 2, 2015.

[17]Stanford Medicine. Available at: http://med.stanford.edu/news/all-news/2011/01/on-your-mark-get-set-interview.html. Accessed May 3, 2015.

[18]University of Nevada School of Medicine. Available at: http://medicine.nevada.edu/asa/admissions/applicants/selection-factors/applicant-interviews. Accessed May 1, 2015.

[19]UAB School of Medicine. Available at: http://www.uab.edu/medicine/news/latest/item/490-mmi-added-to-admissions-process. Accessed May 4, 2015.

[20]The Globe and Mail. Available at: http://www.theglobeandmail.com/life/interview-20-theres-no-easy-way-to-ace-this-one/article1344084/. Accessed May 3, 2015.

[21]UMass Med Now. Available at: http://www.umassmed.edu/news/news-archives/2013/07/mmi-gives-students-multiple-opportunities-to-shine/. Accessed May 3, 2015.

[22]Reiter H, EvaK, Rosenfeld J, Norman G. Multiple mini interviews predict clerkship and licensing examination performance. *Med Educ* 2007; 41 (4): 378-84.

[23]Rees EL, Hawarden AW, Dent G, Hays R, Bates J, Hassell AB. Evidence regarding the utility of multiple mini-interview (MMI) for selection to undergraduate health programs: A BEME systematic review: BEME Guide No. 37. *Med Teach.* 2016;38(5):443-455. doi:10.3109/0142159X.2016.1158799

[24]Langer T, Ruiz C, Tsai P, et al. Transition to multiple mini interview (MMI) interviewing for medical school admissions. *Perspect Med Educ.* 2020;9(4):229-235. doi:10.1007/s40037-020-00605-0

[25]Cleland J, Chu J, Lim S, Low J, Low-Beer N, Kwek TK. COVID 19: Designing and conducting an online mini-multiple interview (MMI) in a dynamic landscape. *Medical Teacher*. 2020;42(7):776-780. doi:10.1080/0142159X.2020.1762851

[26]Ungtrakul T, Lamlertthon W, Boonchoo B, Auewarakul C. Virtual Multiple Mini-Interview during the COVID-19 Pandemic. *Med Educ*. 2020;54(8):764-765. doi:10.1111/medu.14207

[27]Carroll Turpin MA, Steele K, Matuk-Villazon O, Rowland K, Dayton C, Horn K. Rapid Transition to a Virtual Multiple Mini-Interview Admissions Process: A New Medical School's Experience During the COVID-19 Pandemic. *Acad Med*. Published online May 25, 2021. doi:10.1097/ACM.0000000000004179

Chapter 3

Qualities Assessed by MMI

Rule # 4 Medical schools seek certain qualities in their applicants.

Each MMI station is designed to measure or assess a certain noncognitive quality or skill that the medical school has deemed important in its students and future physicians. At some stations, several qualities may be assessed. A survey of admissions officers, representing 90% of U.S. medical schools, provides insight about the personal qualities most commonly assessed.[1]

Personal Characteristics Assessed During the Admissions Interview	
Personal characteristics	**Percentage**
Motivation for a medical career	98%
Compassion and empathy	96%
Personal maturity	92%
Oral communication	91%
Service orientation	89%
Professionalism	88%
Altruism	83%
Integrity	82%
Leadership	80%
Intellectual curiosity	76%
Teamwork	74%
Cultural competence	72%
Reliability and dependability	70%
Self-discipline	70%
Critical thinking	69%
Adaptability	67%
Verbal reasoning	66%
Work habits	66%
Persistence	65%
Resilience	65%
Logical reasoning	56%

Adapted from the AAMC. Available at https://www.aamc.org/download/261110/data/aibvol11_no7.pdf.

Rule # 5   **Ascertain qualities important to the school where you will be interviewing**

How can you tell which of these qualities will be measured during your MMI? Unless you are privy to inside information, you can't know for sure. In fact, medical schools have applicants sign a Participant Agreement and Statement of Confidentiality preventing release or disclosure of MMI information to others. However, a review of the school's website can give you an idea of what is considered important, as shown below for U.S. and Canadian medical schools.

UNITED STATES

ALABAMA

University of Alabama: "We are looking for applicants who have a demonstrated commitment to becoming physicians evidenced by maturing insights into the doctor-patient relationship and a passion for service developed through experiences in a medical setting and through hands on service and volunteer activities; a demonstrated capacity for critical thinking and passion for knowledge..."[2]

ARIZONA

A.T. Still University School of Osteopathic Medicine in Arizona: "As an osteopathic medical school devoted to excellence, we value scholarship, professionalism, learning centeredness, compassion, the whole person (body, mind and spirit), teamwork, and innovation."[3]

University of Arizona: "MMIs...'test' attributes and/or traits sought in a medical student: interpersonal communication, teamwork, ethical and moral judgment, etc."[4]

CALIFORNIA

Stanford University: "...they are simply evaluating interpersonal skills, the ability to communicate clearly, to reason, to be empathic, and so on."[5]

UC Davis: "We're putting our candidates through a series of brief, but telling situations designed to illuminate key characteristic of a good physician, including resourcefulness, listening skills, and even teamwork."[6]

UC Riverside: "The stations and specific prompts used in the MMI process are…evaluating some of the applicants' personal attributes. This core set of criteria includes assessment of the following: a) integrity and ethics, b) reliability and dependability, c) service orientation, d) social and interpersonal skills, e) capacity for improvement, f) resilience and adaptability, g) cultural competence, h) oral communication, and i) teamwork."[7]

Western University of Health Sciences College of Osteopathic Medicine of the Pacific: "I think it helps identify the type of student that would be the best fit for this institution, encompassing the mission that the university has – caring, compassionate, lifelong learners."[8]

ILLINOIS

Chicago Medical School at Rosalind Franklin University of Health and Science: Core values include diversity, innovation, integrity, leadership, professionalism, service, and teamwork.[9]

INDIANA

Marian University College of Osteopathic Medicine: "The format will allow us an opportunity to gauge your non-cognitive skills such as critical thinking and communication—among other areas."[10]

In an interview with The DO, Bryan Moody, Director of Enrollment had this to say about the MMI. "In a physician, you want someone who is going to make good ethical decisions that are sound, taking in vast amounts of information and categorizing it in a way that makes sense to a patient who doesn't have all of that highly scientific knowledge. You want someone who can communicate with you, who can understand and listen and answer questions and speak with you in a way that you can relate to and feel comfortable with. Above all, you want someone who has empathy. Patients come to physicians at their lowest possible moment in life, when they are sick and tired and scared and confused and hurt. And they just want answers."[11]

MASSACHUSETTS

University of Massachusetts: According to Dr. Mariann Manno, Interim Associate Dean, "We want to be able to assess non-cognitive traits such as problem solving, communication, empathy and resilience."[12] UMMS will develop scenarios to measure certain competencies including physician as professional, scientist, communicator, clinical problem solver, patient and community advocate, and person.

MICHIGAN

Central Michigan University: The focus of the 11 stations is on teamwork, ethical and moral dilemmas. Personal and professional attributes considered important include integrity, reliability, positive attitude, adaptability, teamwork, self-discipline, responsibility, compassion, altruism, passion for medicine, communication skills, leadership abilities, personal maturity, and cultural competence.

Michigan State University: "By placing the applicant in a succession of scenarios, we'll be able to test things like a student's resilience, emotional intelligence and a team approach that we can't necessarily appropriately test in the traditional interview process," says Dr. Katherine Ruger, Director of Admissions.[11]

University of Michigan: "You'll have the opportunity to take part in a series of six, six-minute short-form interviews with a variety of people from our med school community. These interactive scenarios will challenge you to demonstrate how you work as part of team, how you think and respond to questions about an ethical or philosophical dilemma, and how you might interact with a patient in a difficult situation—all under a tight time constraint."[13]

Western Michigan University: Personal attributes considered important include teamwork, problem-solving, compassion and dedication to serve others, effective communications, and making decisions with integrity.

MISSOURI

University of Missouri – Kansas City: "...to develop the skills, knowledge, and attitudes of these students longitudinally over six years with a goal of instilling the highest standards of medical professionalism, clinical competency, humanism, and altruism during a highly formative period of their lives."[14]

MISSISSIPPI

University of Mississippi: "The station scenarios do not test or assess scientific or clinical knowledge; instead, they focus on personal competencies such as oral communication skills, service orientation, respect for others including compassion and empathy, critical thinking and decision making, teamwork, awareness of ethics, maturity, coping skills and opinions on health care issues."[15]

NEVADA

University of Nevada: "Each station is designed to assess applicant communication skills, ability to solve problems and think critically, and ethics and integrity."[16]

NEW JERSEY

UMDNJ – Robert Wood Johnson Medical School: "The stations may be comprised of scenarios which do not test or assess scientific knowledge but will focus on issues such as communication, ethics, service, critical thinking and adaptability."[17]

NEW YORK

New York Medical College: "…interpersonal skills, communication, professionalism, cultural competency, and teamwork are paramount."[18]

New York University: "Scenarios may explore an applicant's communication skills, ability to work as part of a team, problem solving capabilities, integrity, ethics and judgment."[19]

SUNY Upstate Medical University: "We drive innovation and discovery by empowering our university family to bring forth new ideas and to ensure quality. We respect people by treating all with grace and dignity and embracing diversity. We serve our community by living our mission. We value integrity by being open and honest to build trust and teamwork."[20]

OHIO

University of Cincinnati: "Because physicians need good communication, critical thinking, and teamwork skills, we are very interested in evaluating these characteristics in our applicants."[21]

OKLAHOMA

University of Oklahoma College of Medicine: "These are our core values: We believe that caring for our patients must be at the center of all we do. We act with honesty and integrity. We respect our colleagues and co-workers. We magnify our effectiveness through teamwork. We improve continually through harnessing innovation and encouraging high performance. We believe in open and effective communication. We are committed to providing outstanding educational programs. We will be a leader in the advancement of basic, translational and clinical research. We embrace our social responsibilities with pride."[22]

OREGON

Oregon Health & Science University: "Attributes that enhance team-based health care, like communication skills, comfort with mutual decision-making and respect for other health professionals will be increasingly important. The MMI process will help in our ongoing goal to always be educating the types of physicians most needed by society."[23]

UTAH

University of Utah School of Medicine: "Interviewers will explore the applicant's motivation for seeking a medical degree, awareness and understanding of the medical profession, leadership, problem solving skills, understanding of medical ethics and interpersonal skills."[24]

VERMONT

University of Vermont College of Medicine: "The goal, says UVM College of Medicine Associate Dean of Admissions Jan Gallant, M.D., is to assess a student's readiness for medical school through the lens of the core personal competencies identified by the Association for American Medical Colleges (AAMC). These competencies include ethical responsibility, a capacity for improvement, cultural competence and adaptability."[25]

VIRGINIA

Virginia Tech University Carilion School of Medicine: "In the MMI process, each interviewer will pose a pre-developed scenario to each interviewee related to a single theme (such as 'Professionalism /Interdisciplinary Teamwork')…The MMI can also assess the applicant's ability to function in team settings, an important skill for our small group learning curriculum."[26]

WASHINGTON

Pacific Northwest University of Health Sciences College of Osteopathic Medicine: "Our initial College of Osteopathic Medicine has a mission to train compassionate and competent osteopathic physicians to fill the health care needs in the Pacific Northwest, especially in rural and medically underserved areas…Institutional values include mission driven (committed to create, sustain, and improve quality educational programs specifically for rural and medically underserved communities), collaborative (working together with thoughtful actions, efforts, and concerns to meet each opportunity, issue, or challenge presented), compassionate (every individual is respected and treated with consideration, kindness, and understanding), and genuine (real people providing real solutions which have direct impact on community health, resources, and outcomes)."[27]

CANADA

ALBERTA

University of Alberta Faculty of Medicine: "The questions will be designed to evaluate the interviewee's critical thinking abilities, ethical decision-making abilities, communication skills and overall performance."[28]

University of Calgary Faculty of Medicine: Seeks students who will demonstrate attributes of altruism, compassion, empathy, and integrity. Also valued are honesty, respect for others, confidentiality, self-directed learning, strong work ethic, and communication skills. "The University of Calgary aims to admit students who will demonstrate ability to manage time, tolerate ambiguity and stress, good judgment, enthusiasm for their work, pay attention to detail, and recognize and respect the roles of other healthcare disciplines."[29]

BRITISH COLUMBIA

University of British Columbia Faculty of Medicine: "The UBC MMI is designed to see how you think on your feet, how you communicate what you believe when pondering ethical, moral and other dilemmas (which are not necessarily medically-related), and to explore who you are as a person."[30]

MANITOBA

University of Manitoba Faculty of Medicine: The institution seeks students who are open to practicing medicine in urban hubs and rural parts of Canada. Also important is an emphasis on "healing through knowledge and compassion and acting as educators for patients, allied health professionals, and one another." Other points of emphasis include effective communication with other professionals, professionalism, respect, cultural safety, and compassionate care to diverse patient populations.[31]

NEWFOUNDLAND

Memorial University of Newfoundland Faculty of Medicine: "The Admissions Committee seeks in applicants the same humanistic qualities and attitudes that our medical school considers essential in a physician: integrity, a respect for others' choices and rights, compassion, empathy, personal insight, ability to communicate effectively and relate to people, maturity and motivation."[32]

NOVA SCOTIA

Dalhousie University Faculty of Medicine: "The stations are designed to assess the applicant's personal qualities, such as problem solving, thinking on your feet, leading, balance, compassion, motivation, critical thinking, awareness of societal health issues, communication skills and ethics."[33]

ONTARIO

McMaster University Michael G. DeGroote School of Medicine: "The stations deal with a variety of issues, which may include but are not limited to, communication, collaboration, ethics, health policy, critical thinking, awareness of society health issues in Canada and personal qualities."[34]

Northern Ontario School of Medicine: The school seeks students who will be socially accountable to the needs of the population in northern Ontario, including Aboriginal, Francophone, remote, rural, and underserviced communities. Values prized include innovation, social accountability, collaboration, inclusiveness, and respect.[35]

Queen's University Faculty of Health Sciences: "The goal of using the MMI is to more effectively assess non-cognitive qualities of an applicant, which could include empathy, critical thinking, ethical decision making and communication skills."[36]

QUEBEC

McGill University Faculty of Medicine: Qualities valued include compassion, empathy, insight, judgment, honesty, adaptability, tolerance, creativity, respect for others, intellectual curiosity, reliability, teamwork, conflict or stress management, leadership, initiative, self-confidence, and professionalism.[37]

SASKATCHEWAN

University of Saskatchewan: "Station scenarios may be structured to specifically judge a candidate's ethical and critical decision-making abilities, knowledge of the health-care system, understanding of health determinants in a local or global context, commitment to helping others, non-academic achievements, or desire for studying medicine."[38]

References

[1]Dunleavy D, Whittaker K. The evolving medical school admissions interview. *AIB* 2011; 11 (7).
[2]UAB School of Medicine. Available at: http://www.uab.edu/medicine/home/future-students/admissions/welcome. Accessed May 3, 2015.
[3]School of Osteopathic Medicine in Arizona. Available at: https://www.atsu.edu/soma/about/mission.htm. Accessed May 4, 2015.
[4]University of Arizona College of Medicine. Available at: http://medicine.arizona.edu/alumni/alumni-slide/tucson-admissions-implements-new-interview-technique. Accessed May 4, 2015.
[5]Stanford Medicine. Available at: http://med.stanford.edu/news/all-news/2011/11/5-questions-prober-on-new-approach-to-admission-interviews.html. Accessed January 2, 2015.
[6]UC Davis Health System. Available at: http://www.ucdmc.ucdavis.edu/publish/news/newsroom/4447. Accessed May4, 2015.
[7]University of California Riverside School of Medicine. Available at: http://www.ucop.edu/operating-budget/_files/legreports/1314/progressreportucr-somlegrpt-4-2-14.pdf. Accessed May 3, 2015.
[8]Western University of Health Sciences. Available at: http://jprod.westernu.edu/news/nr_detail.jsp?id=13243. Accessed May 4, 2015.
[9]Rosalind Franklin University of Health and Science. Available at: http://www.rosalindfranklin.edu/Degreeprograms/corevalues.aspx. Accessed May 4, 2015.
[10]Marian University College of Osteopathic Medicine. Available at: http://www.marian.edu/osteopathic-medical-school/interview. Accessed May 4, 2015.
[11]The DO. Available at: http://thedo.osteopathic.org/2014/09/multple-mini-interviews-gains-traction-schools/. Accessed May 4, 2015.
[12]UMass Med Now. Available at: http://www.umassmed.edu/news/news-archives/2013/07/mmi-gives-students-multiple-opportunities-to-shine/. Accessed May 4, 2015.
[13]University of Michigan Medical School. Available at: http://medicine.umich.edu/medschool/education/md-program/md-admissions/interview-day/faqs. Accessed May 4, 2015.
[14]UMKC School of Medicine. Available at: http://med.umkc.edu/about_us/vision-goals/. Accessed May 4, 2015.
[15]University of Mississippi Medical Center. Available at: http://www.umc.edu/Education/Schools/Medicine/SOM_Admissions/Interviews.aspx. Accessed May 4, 2015.
[16]University of Nevada School of Medicine. Available at: http://medicine.nevada.edu/asa/admissions/applicants/selection-factors/applicant-interviews. Accessed May 4, 2015.
[17]Robert Wood Johnson Medical School. Available at: http://rwjms.rutgers.edu/education/admissions/selection_process.html. Accessed May 4, 2015.
[18]New York Medical College InTouch. Available at: http://www.nymc.edu/OfficesAndServices/PublicRelations/Assets/June2012_InTouch.pdf. Accessed May 4, 2015.
[19]NYU School of Medicine. Available at: https://www.med.nyu.edu/school/md-admissions/mmi-faqs. Accessed May 4, 2015.
[20]State University of New York Upstate Medical University. Available at: http://www.upstate.edu/excellence/pdf/values.pdf. Accessed May 4, 2015.
[21]University of Cincinnati College of Medicine. Available at: http://healthnews.uc.edu/news/?/14446/. Accessed May 4, 2015.

[22]University of Oklahoma College of Medicine. Available at:
http://www.oumedicine.com/collegeofmedicine. Accessed May 4, 2015.
[23]Oregon Health & Science University. Available at:
http://www.ohsu.edu/xd/education/schools/school-of-medicine/about/school-of-medicine-news/education-news/multiple-mini-interviews-4111.cfm. Accessed May 4, 2015.
[24]University of Utah School of Medicine. Available at:
http://medicine.utah.edu/admissions/process/. Accessed May 4, 2015.
[25]University of Vermont College of Medicine. Available at:
http://www.uvm.edu/medicine/?Page=news&storyID=19920&category=comall. Accessed May 4, 2015.
[26]Virginia Tech Carilion School of Medicine. Available at:
http://www.vtc.vt.edu/education/admissions/interview_day.html. Accessed May 4, 2015.
[27]Pacific Northwest University of Health Sciences College of Osteopathic Medicine. Available at: http://www.pnwu.edu/assets/PDFs/Student-Catalog/2014-2015-Student-CatalogFinal-Contentv2.pdf. Accessed March 2, 2015.
[28]University of Alberta Faculty of Medicine. Available at:
https://www.med.ualberta.ca/programs/md/admissions/applying/interview. Accessed May 15, 2015.
[29]University of Calgary Faculty of Medicine. Available at:
http://www.ucalgary.ca/mdprogram/admissions/mmi-information. Accessed May 12, 2015.
[30]University of British Columbia Faculty of Medicine. Available at:
http://mdprogram.med.ubc.ca/admissions/interviews/. Accessed May 12, 2015.
[31]University of Manitoba Faculty of Medicine. Available at:
http://umanitoba.ca/faculties/health_sciences/medicine/education/undergraduate/ugme_mission_objectives.html. Accessed May 12, 2015.
[32]Memorial University of Newfoundland Faculty of Medicine. Available at:
http://www.med.mun.ca/Admissions/ApplicationEvaluationCompetitions.aspx. Accessed May 12, 2015.
[33]Dalhousie University Faculty of Medicine. Available at:
http://medicine.dal.ca/departments/core-units/admissions/application-process/interview.html. Accessed May 12, 2015.
[34]McMaster University Michael G. DeGroote School of Medicine. Available at:
http://fhs.mcmaster.ca/mdprog/interviews.html. Accessed May 12, 2015.
[35]Northern Ontario School of Medicine. Available at:
http://www.medicaleducationfutures.org/sites/default/files/Beyond%20Flexer%20NOSM%20Final%20Report.pdf. Accessed May 12, 2015.
[36]Queen's University Faculty of Health Sciences. Available at:
http://meds.queensu.ca/education/undergraduate/prospective_students/application_process/interview. Accessed May 12, 2015.
[37]McGill University Faculty of Medicine. Available at:
http://www.mcgill.ca/medadmissions/applying/selection-process/message-applicants. Accessed May 12, 2015.
[38]University of Saskatchewan College of Medicine. Available at:
http://www.medicine.usask.ca/education/medical/undergrad/prospective-students/admissions/MMI%20Fact%20Sheet.pdf. Accessed May 12, 2015.

Chapter 4

MMI Format

Rule # 6   **Become familiar with the MMI format**

During the MMI, the interviewee moves from one station to another over about a two-hour period. At each station, the interviewee is asked to respond to one of the following:

- Short structured scenario
- Question
- Task

Trained raters (interviewers) are present to observe and score the candidate's performance. Applicants will receive the same question, scenario, or task, and this allows raters to easily compare the quality of responses among a group of candidates.

Typical MMI Format

- The typical MMI involves 8 to 10 stations.

- You'll be presented with various scenarios, usually posted on the door.

- You'll have 2 minutes to read each scenario.

- You may or may not be able to take notes.

- You'll then be prompted to enter the room, where you will respond to the scenario or task.

SEQUENCE OF EVENTS DURING MMI STATION

*The process continues until the applicant has completed all stations.

Rule # 7   **Recognize the differences between the major types of MMI stations**

There will be three main types of MMI stations you will encounter as an interviewee. These station types along with representative examples are shown below.

Question/Discussion Station

Upon entering the room, you will likely find yourself with one rater (interviewer). You will respond to the prompt, and the rater may then ask you follow-up questions. These follow-up questions will differ from one applicant to another, depending on the content of the initial response.

Question stations are designed to assess communication skills, thought processes, and professionalism.

Question/Discussion Station Examples

Dr. Cheung recommends homeopathic medicines to his patients. There is no scientific evidence or widely accepted theory to suggest that homeopathic medicines work, and Dr. Cheung doesn't believe them to. He recommends homeopathic medicine to people with mild and nonspecific symptoms such a fatigue, headaches and muscle aches, because he believes that it will do no harm, but will give them reassurance. Consider the ethical problems that Dr. Cheung's behavior might pose. Discuss these issues with the interviewer.[1]

Recently in Congress, there has been a discussion concerning the issue of deterrent fees for all individuals on either Medicare or Medicaid (a small charge, say $20), which everyone who initiates a visit to a health professional would have to pay for every contact as a way to control health care costs. The assumption is that this will deter people from visiting their doctor for unnecessary reasons. Consider the broad implications of this policy for health and health care costs. For example, do you think the approach will save health care costs? At what expense?[2]

Another type of question station focuses on either traditional interview questions or behavioral interview questions. The traditional interview questions (as the name states) are the classic medical school interview questions. These include questions such as "why do you want to become a physician?" and "why did you apply to our medical school?" Behavioral interview questions, in contrast, delve into your previous behavior. "Tell me about a time when you had a conflict with a colleague."

Scenario/Acting Station

Prior to entering the room, you will be given a scenario to read. Inside the room, you'll find two people – rater and actor. The actor has been trained to engage in the scenario with you. The rater will observe your interactions with the actor. Scenario stations often provide information about an applicant's compassion, social interaction, and problem solving.

Scenario/Acting Station Examples

The parking garage at your place of work has assigned parking spots. On leaving your spot, you are observed by the garage attendant as you back into a neighboring car, a BMW, knocking out its left front headlight and denting the left front fender. The garage attendant gives you the name and office number of the owner of the neighboring car, telling you that he is calling ahead to the car owner, Tim. The garage attendant tells you that Tim is expecting your visit. Enter Tim's office.[1]

You have a meeting set up with Frankie. He is the son of a family friend who moved to Thunder Bay about 20 years ago and so you have never met him. He has come down from Thunder Bay to look over "southern universities." He urgently needs some information on schools as he will have to make some serious decisions soon. He is happy to get this meeting as he realizes how tight your schedule is. In fact, your next meeting is in eight minutes. Frankie is in the room.[3]

Task/Collaboration Station

You will be asked to complete a task, often with another applicant. The Stanford University School of Medicine offers the following description of a task station:[2]

Two applicants participate in a scenario in which one applicant is asked to perform a complex test (such as assembling or repairing a model) with the other applicant giving directions for dealing with or assembling the model.

When you enter the room, there will be two raters, one of whom will be responsible for observing and rating your performance. The second rater will be tasked with evaluating the other applicant. Task stations are used to learn more about an applicant's teamwork, problem solving, and communication skills.

Task/Collaboration Station Example

Origami (Deliver): When you enter the room there will be a sheet of paper that illustrates how to complete an origami (paper folding) project. On the other side of the room there is another candidate who can't look at you, but who has a blank piece of paper. Verbally guide your colleague to completion of the origami project.[3]

Origami (Receive): When you enter the room there will be a blank sheet of paper in front of you. On the other side of the room there is another candidate who will provide you with instructions regarding how to turn this page into an origami (paper folding) project. Do not look at the other candidate until told to do so.[3]

Rule # 8   **The MMI interview will differ from one school to another. Try to learn the details of the MMI at the school where you'll be interviewing.**

Although the basic structure of the MMI will be similar, there may be differences with respect to:

- Duration of MMI session
- Number of stations
- Duration of encounter at each station
- Number of rest breaks
- Note-taking

Acquiring this information in advance of the interview day will allow you to adjust your preparation and mindset accordingly. Begin with the school's website and written correspondence. You can also contact the school for more information. Schools may share this information if you ask. This approach will help you avoid common pitfalls:

- I remember one applicant who had interviewed at a school where interviewees were given 8 minutes to address the question, task, or scenario at each station. She assumed that she would be given the same chunk of time at her next MMI interview. On the day of her interview, she was thrown for a loop when the school informed her that she would have only 5 minutes per station.

- Another applicant was surprised to learn that she wouldn't be able to jot down notes during the two minutes she had before entering the room. This school's policy was a departure from the MMIs she had taken part in at two other schools. She struggled to adapt, and felt that her answers lacked structure and organization.

Did you know...

If the medical school's website does not provide details about the logistics or structure of the MMI, ask the admissions office for this information. Admissions offices may provide an overview of the interview day and details about the MMI format. "A week in advance, we e-mail applicants detailed instructions explaining how our MMI works," said Gurmeet Rai, Manager of the Office of Education at UC Davis.[4]

Did you know...

You may be wondering how schools develop their MMI scenarios. In some cases, these scenarios are licensed from other institutions like McMaster University, where the MMI was founded. Schools may also rely on faculty and students for development. "Each year faculty, students and community members are invited to assist with developing scenarios for the interview process...Once the interview process is complete, you will be informed whether or not your scenario was selected for use. Those chosen will be awarded a $ 50 honorarium."[10]

Admissions Officers Speak...

"The MMI is a series of 8 interview stations consisting of timed interview scenarios. Applicants rotate through the stations, each with its own interviewer and scenario. The MMI session lasts approximately 72 minutes."[5]

New York University School of Medicine

"There will be a two-minute break between each station. The MMI session lasts approximately 100 minutes. Yes, you will have at least one to two rest breaks during your MMI session."[6]

Michigan State University College of Human Medicine

"You will interact with the interviewers for seven minutes. You will be informed when time is up. There will be a two minute break between stations. The MMI itself, including all the mini-interview stations, lasts approximately 90 minutes."[7]

University of Arizona College of Medicine

"The MMI is a series of approximately six to eight interview 'stations' or encounters that last eight to 10 minutes and are centered on a scenario. Each station has its own interviewer (rater); consequently, each student is evaluated by approximately six to eight different individuals."[8]

University of Cincinnati College of Medicine

"Applicants will participate in each MMI station for seven minutes. Students are informed when time is up. There will be a one-minute break between stations."[9]

University of Nevada School of Medicine

As I write this in 2021, we know that many medical school interviews will be held virtually. Although traditional interviews are challenging, virtual interviews introduce a whole new set of challenges and a new level of complexity.

Will medical school interviews be virtual for the 2021-2022 application cycle?

Many medical schools will be using a virtual or "remote" interview format for the 2021-2022 application cycle.

- Medical schools announcing the use of remote interviews for this cycle include the Pritzker School of Medicine at UChicago, the Emory School of Medicine, and many others.
- Since the situation is constantly evolving, we encourage you to look into specific schools and prepare for their interview formats.
- For more information about interview procedures for different medical schools in the 2021-2022 application cycle, please see this resource, available online from the AAMC: Medical School Admission Requirements™ (MSAR®) Report for Applicants and Advisors: Interview Procedures 2022.

What should I expect from a virtual medical school interview?

In this section, we're focusing on recommendations for a traditional interview and MMI questions. You might also be asked to participate in other formats during virtual interviews.

- Some schools in 2020 used breakout rooms to help administer virtual MMI interviews.
- Other applicants have participated in virtual group interviews, which may introduce their own challenges.
- In group interviews, one interviewer speaks to a group of applicants at the same time, interviewing the entire group at once. (You can imagine how stressful that might be: applicants hesitant to speak, others speaking over each other...)

The strategies below will be useful for all types of virtual interviews. Our best advice if you'll be facing specific interview variations is to be familiar with the different interview formats.

Although your interview prep for both in-person and virtual interviews will be similar, there are some unique features of the virtual interview that you need to take into account.

This section outlines seven strategies for preparing for virtual interviews

Virtual interviews are stressful. Period. From the vagaries of technology to the importance of virtual first impressions, there's a lot to consider. That's why we developed seven strategies for preparing for virtual interviews.

These cover the basics of what an applicant should do to succeed in their interview, from the moment they first receive a virtual interview invitation to the day of the interview itself.

- In this section, we'll highlight how to prepare for the virtual interview.
- In the next section, we'll be highlighting expert recommendations on how to succeed on the actual day of your virtual interview.

I just received an invitation for a virtual interview. What do I do now?

Strategy #1: Read Your Interview Invitation Carefully

Your interview invitation has several key pieces of information that are crucial for your planning and preparation. This is why it's important to read the email you received from the program very carefully.

This is what you need to look for in your virtual interview email invite:
1. Your interview time
2. The interview day schedule

3. The timings of each event that will take place during that day
4. Which platform the interview will be conducted on (e.g. Zoom, Skype, Google, or another video conferencing platform)

Once you know what platform will be used, you can start taking steps to become technologically ready for the interview.

Check your email regularly to make sure there haven't been any changes to your interview invitations

How to Become Technologically Ready: The Importance of Back-up Devices and Strong Internet Connections

Being technologically ready means taking steps to prepare yourself and your devices so that your virtual interview proceeds as smoothly as possible. The next few strategies focus on technological readiness, since the reliance on technology is one of the largest differences between virtual and in-person interviews.

Your best interview responses will fail to make an impact if your technology fails you. Having conducted hundreds of virtual interviews, I've found that technological issues happen often. This can certainly affect the impression that applicants make on interviewers.

If you've never experienced a technology failure, lucky you. We've experienced these ourselves multiple times. Dr. Katta is a frequent media contributor through her work with the American Academy of Dermatology and relayed this anecdote:

I was getting ready to interview with a CBS News Producer. I am definitely familiar with the major platforms, but then I ran into an issue with the camera app on my laptop. It turns out that it was interfering with my webcam. I figured it out in time, but racing against the clock to try to decipher my computer issues did not help my stress levels. Especially with my stress levels already high enough in the five minutes prior to being "on-air."

One thing that helped control her anxiety was that she had a laptop, a desktop, and a phone with the platform app all ready to go. If she hadn't figured out her laptop issue in time, she was ready to head to her desktop.

Having those backup devices ready to go is critical.

Strategy #2: Keep a Backup Device Ready in Case of Emergency

It's important to have multiple devices prepared. When it comes to technology, you can never really be sure of what might happen.

Most applicants use a laptop as their primary device. But you have to ask yourself: what happens if my laptop breaks down during the interview?

While you might think this is a remote possibility, I can say from doing virtual interviews that I've seen this happen to a fair share of applicants. Hence, I always tell people to have a second device ready to go as their backup.

Take these steps to make sure that both your primary and secondary devices are technologically ready:

- Have the most up-to-date version of the video conferencing platform installed on both devices.
- Test your audio and video to make sure your equipment is linked and compatible with the software.

Preparing multiple devices for your virtual interview is one of the best steps you can take to ensure your interview proceeds smoothly--even if you experience technical difficulties.

Strategy #3: Secure a Strong Internet Connection

Every video conferencing platform will have recommendations for optimal internet speed. You can do your own speed test on your internet connection to ensure that it meets these optimal speeds by using websites such as fast.com.

Questions to keep in mind:

- Is my internet speed sufficient?
- Does my internet speed exceed what is recommended by the video conferencing program?
- Have I experienced any issues with internet speed or video conferencing at this location in the past?
- Does my internet speed differ from room to room?
- Are other people nearby using Wi-Fi?
- Should I consider using Ethernet for my interview instead?

There are times when your home won't be the best place to have your virtual interview. If your connection speed is an issue, for example, I've had applicants do their interviews from their library, university, or even a hotel.

If you choose to do your interview elsewhere, <u>practice in that location</u> before your interview. The more practice at the actual interview location, the better. You'll feel more comfortable and it's less likely that you'll encounter surprises.

One of our students, Jenny, recalls her Wi-Fi failing during a virtual interview. Five minutes into the interview, the call dropped. Eventually, Jenny contacted the interviewer and conducted the rest of the interview using data on her cell phone.

Testing Wi-Fi speeds and keeping a backup device can be vital in ensuring your virtual interview experience is as stress-free as possible.

Strategy #4: Be Intentional with Your Background

You need to remember that when your interview starts, your interviewer is already forming an impression of you. Much of this is subconscious. Some of that first impression will be formed from your environment, specifically your background.

Consider the presentation of your background:

- How much will the interviewer see behind you?
- Is your background cluttered or disorganized?

- What do you have hanging on the wall or sitting on your bookshelf?
- What does the content of your background imply about you?

Some of our students have considered this, and have taken steps to intentionally "design" their background:

- Several have interviewed in front of bookshelves or display shelving
- Some students might choose to display something relevant to themselves or their interests in their background, as a way to garner intrigue or start a conversation.
- One student reported placing some of her artwork in the background to display her hobby.
- If you decide to use a virtual background, such as the preset options on Zoom, make sure it looks professional and works with your lighting.
- If all else fails, I tell applicants there's nothing wrong with having a blank wall behind them.

I think this is going to be a really interesting area of research in the future, because we just don't have a lot of research yet on how applicants are judged during virtual interviews.

Having said that, we have done a lot of writing and reading on the subject of first impressions, and we frequently speak about proper interview attire and careful grooming. These are subconscious impressions and form quickly. I think your interview background may be considered in a similar way.

Let me be clear here: I don't think an interviewer would *say*, "I noticed your room is messy." Instead, they might take it in as a subconscious impression.

One way to think about this topic is to consider that your interview background is essentially an extension of your interview attire. Remember that your background will form an important part of your first impression.

Strategy #5: Choose Your Chair Wisely

Yes, you heard me right. Pay attention to your chair. Why? Because posture is a key component of non-verbal communication.

Your posture contributes to first impressions and overall impressions. While your posture may be off for a variety of reasons, one variable you can control is the type of chair you're sitting in.

Applicants may not realize this ahead of time, but often you'll be sitting in this chair for hours straight. While some programs provide breaks in between each event or interview, some of my students have told me that they didn't get any breaks for five hours. Imagine that for just a moment. You might be sitting in a chair for five hours straight. Hence, you need to have a comfortable chair that helps support good posture.

Beyond comfort, make sure your chair isn't overly distracting to yourself or the interviewer. This means taking into consideration how much your chair swivels, leans back, or makes noise when you move.

Strategy #6: Make sure that everyone around you knows that you have an important interview

I tell applicants to keep the people in their life informed. This serves both a social and a logistical purpose. With most applicants doing virtual interviews at home, there are often others present.

Applicants usually do a good job of making sure they're not disturbed by the people with whom they live. But sometimes they don't realize how much noise can seep through, even with the door closed.

Have that talk with the members of your household about keeping noise to a minimum.

Strategy #7: Prepare for the Unexpected

We can do everything right on our end. And then, despite our best efforts, technology fails us. This can happen not only to individual applicants--it can also affect medical schools and programs. In the face of technology failure, how you handle the situation is critical.

This is why it's so important to prepare for the unexpected. (I would have said "prepare for the unthinkable", except that technology failures are surprisingly common.)

- Several days before the interview, email the admissions office or program coordinator of the residency program
- In this email, state that you are looking forward to the interview
- Confirm your interview date and time
- Ask about the best phone number to use in case of technical difficulties
- Some programs include this information in their interview invitations. If they haven't, don't hesitate to reach out.

Especially when it comes to the challenges of technology and the internet, preparation is key.

How to Ensure Success on the Day of Your Virtual Interview

In this section, we explore the steps to take on the day of your interview, to ensure that you're prepared to deliver your best interview performance. There are a number of factors that are unique to virtual interviews, so it's important to be aware of these factors and prepared for them. These 5 expert strategies can help.

Strategy #1: Make Sure Distractions Don't Detract From Your Interview Performance

There are plenty of potential distractions, especially if you're interviewing from home.

- First of all, make sure you've informed everyone with whom you share your interview space with about the date, time, and duration of your interview in advance.
- The day of, consider placing a note on your door as a reminder.
- If your Wi-Fi speeds vary based on how many people are using it nearby, consider reminding your household members of this again the day of the interview.

Other Possible Interview Distractions and How to Avoid Them

Walk through your space and just listen for a moment. Now think about how this space might sound during the course of a day. What types of sounds and distractions might you encounter on a typical day? These may include:

- Doorbells
- A landline phone
- Cell phone ringer and vibrations
- Alerts on your desktop
- Cooking and kitchen noises
- Lawnmower
- Construction sounds

I remember interviewing one applicant and then, right in the middle of a heartfelt response, the doorbell rang. It threw this poor applicant completely off his game.

That's why I recommend this tactic: Cover the doorbell and put a note up on the front door. "Please do not ring the doorbell or knock on the door. Job interview is in progress."

Along those same lines, I always ask applicants if they have a landline phone. I know that's becoming less common, but if you do, you certainly don't want that phone to ring. I tell applicants to shut off the ringer.

Something else to note is outside noise. If you have a lawn service, you want to make sure they don't show up the day of your interview. For people who live in colder locations, it might be a snowblower.

Another distraction is computer alerts. I think many of us have become immune to these noises, but they can be very distracting to your interviewer. Turn off those notifications on your computer. When I first started podcasting, it didn't take me long to realize I had overlooked my desktop alerts: as soon as I listened to the tape, I realized just how much noise my desktop produced.

Strategy #2: Optimize the Lighting in Your Space

Lighting is huge, and I think applicants don't factor this in as much as they should. I've worked with applicants not only from the US but from other countries as well. These virtual interviews are going to be taking place at US time, either in the morning or afternoon.

- I recommend that you record yourself at different points of the day to see how you look.
- Make sure that you have the appropriate lighting.
- If you're in a room with a window, think about how the light from the window affects the lighting where you're going to be sitting. The look of light can vary depending on the time of the day. I personally like to set up in front of an open window so that the light from the window is shining on my face.
- Avoid sitting in a location where the light is coming from behind you---you will be backlit and the interviewer will not see your face properly.
- I have to say one of the best devices I've purchased was a ring light that I purchased from Amazon. Note that it doesn't work the best if you have glasses (due to an annoying reflection on your lenses). Apart from that, it produces a nice even glow to your face.
- Although I don't think this is necessary, several webcams allow you to adjust for lighting on the screen. If you'll be doing several virtual interviews, you may decide to invest in one of these handy devices.

Here's Dr. Katta's take on lighting:

Last year I was on a video conference call with participants from Paris. The meeting was scheduled for very early in the morning, and I had no natural light. To prepare, I took a lot of photographs to see how I looked with my artificial light source. It definitely took a lot of experimentation to determine the best location for my light source.

If you have the option, my favorite source is still natural light from a big window in front of me. My next favorite option is having that additional ring light shine on my face.

Try different lighting set-ups to see what suit you the most. Having interviewers be able to see your face clearly is obviously important.

Strategy #3: Think About Your Equipment and Accessories

What do I do with my cell phone?

Some applicants will shut off their cell phones. What I tell them is that I'd rather them not shut off their cell phone. You never know when the medical school or residency program will need to reach out to you. Programs will try to do that via the phone. For example, technological issues not only affect applicants-they can also affect the medical school or residency program.

- Keep your phone near you
- Silence your phone
- If the program has technical difficulties, be ready for a call from them
- If you have technical difficulties, you'll have your phone close by to call the program

Keep These Other Items Close By During Your Interview

- Writing utensils: You need to have multiple writing utensils accessible to you. I've done virtual interviews where the applicant's pen runs dry and they tell me to hold on for a minute while they grab a replacement. Remember: If you wouldn't do it during an in-person interview, you don't want to do it during a virtual interview.

- Notepad: Having a notepad is also recommended so that you can take notes. On interview days, you won't just be answering questions. You'll have an orientation session, perhaps one in which the Dean or the program director spends time discussing the particular aspects of their program.

- Water bottle: These interviews can stretch on to be fairly full days---and you'll be doing a lot of talking. Having a water bottle handy can help.

Strategy #4:
Remember the Importance and the Impact of Nonverbal Communication

Let's talk about how nonverbal impressions send a message to the interviewer. A lot of applicants focus mainly (or exclusively) on the content of their answers and they don't realize how important those nonverbal aspects of their answers are.

In my books *The Successful Match* and *The Medical School Interview*, I review the effects of nonverbal impressions on in-person interviews. Although this hasn't been researched as extensively in virtual interviews, the same lessons should apply.

Avoid Nervous Habits or Tics

In thinking about body language, you want to make sure that you don't default to nervous habits or tics when you're under stress. I've seen it all during interviews.

During your practice interviews, make sure your partner informs of you of any of nervous habits. Examples include:

- Finger tapping
- Rapid blinking
- Nervous laughter
- Pen tapping
- Pen twirling
- Hair swirling
- And more

The importance of maintaining eye contact during a virtual interview

Poor eye contact is one of the most common mistakes that I see in virtual interviews. The natural tendency when you're in a virtual interview is to look at the interviewer's face, similarly to an in-person interview.

However, there's an important consideration here. When you look at the interviewer's face in a virtual interview, they see you as looking down. They don't see you as looking at them and making good eye contact. This is a result of the camera being at the center top of your computer and the interviewer's face being several inches below the camera.

This results in a major issue. According to research, eye contact is crucial to the impression you give to interviewers. When you fail to make eye contact with an interviewer, you communicate a different message, which may be that:

- You aren't interested in what they're saying
- You are a poor listener
- You are not engaged in the conversation
- You have something to hide

To avoid this issue, I've started minimizing my browser and moving that person's face as close to my laptop camera as I can. That way I can be partially looking at their face but still mainly looking at the camera. I've also given a presentation where I had to speak directly to the camera, which took practice.

The Importance of Good Posture and a Good Chair

You have to factor in whether the chair you're using could affect your body language. For example, some individuals use chairs that recline, swivel, or have wheels. During virtual interviews, some people are moving back and forth due to the recliner or the swivel action of that chair. This can be very distracting for interviewers--and applicants often don't realize this is happening.

I've also seen applicants reclining in their comfortable chairs, not realizing that this may come off as disinterest, apathy, or low energy.

I wrote earlier about the importance of choosing a good, comfortable chair for interviews. Definitely make sure you've planned ahead. A chair that doesn't easily move or rock and that allows you to maintain a good posture is important.

Strategy #5: Plan Ahead For Technical Difficulties

What if I have a technological problem in the middle of an interview?

In our previous section about preparing for virtual interviews, we recommended securing the phone number to contact the medical school or residency program in case of tech issues.

If you do encounter technical difficulties during your interview, remember to:

- Stay calm and composed
- Know that programs and schools are understanding when it comes to technological issues. These are frequent occurrences.
- Maintain your composure, since you will be judged on how you react to this stressful situation

Common Questions

Should I have Post-It notes with interview tips or questions for the interviewer?

I've had applicants ask this question, and it's a good one. Unfortunately, if you have notes that are taped or accessible on your computer, it does create a potential problem. Primarily, this can take your gaze away from the camera, which affects your eye contact.

In mock interviews, I've had applicants ask: "I prepared the answer to that question. Is it okay if I just read that off the screen?" When they've done so, unfortunately it's really easy to tell that they're looking somewhere else.

Apart from eye contact, this also suggests that you're not entirely prepared. Remember, the impression you want to make is that you are 100% prepared for the interview and 100% engaged with the interviewer.

Be confident in your interview skills and maintain eye contact.

Can I have food or drink nearby during the interview?

I don't recommend having food or drink, including coffee, in your background during the interview. Instead, I recommend eating or drinking during breaks.

The one exception to this rule would be if you need a sip of water. If you're in the middle of your interview and you feel that your throat is dry, you can certainly take a sip of water. If you feel the need to do so, you can ask the interviewer, "Dr. Smith, before I answer your question, do you mind if I just take a sip of water?"

Final recommendations

- Put in the time to practice thoroughly
- I highly recommend mock interviews
- Record yourself during the mock interview. Then, with a trusted partner, arrange a time to go through the recorded interview session
- Play the recording and focus on the lighting, the position of your face on the screen, and any nervous habits or mannerisms
- Technology is certainly a factor in virtual interviews. Make sure that technology works for you rather than against you.

References

[1] Eva K, Rosenfeld J, Reiter H, Norman G. An admissions OSCE: the multiple mini-interview. *Med Educ* 2004; 38 (3): 314-26.
[2] Stanford Medicine. Available at: deansnewsletter.stanford.edu/word_docs/DeanNews11-08-10.doc. Accessed May 4, 2015.
[3] Eva K, Reiter H, Rosenfeld J, Norman G. The relationship between interviewers' characteristics and ratings assigned during a multiple-mini interview. *Acad Med* 2004; 79 (6): 602-9.
[4] UC Davis School of Medicine. Available at: https://www.ucdmc.ucdavis.edu/facultydev/pdfs/FacDevNLDec10_Jan11_pages.pdf. Accessed May 29, 2015.
[5] New York University School of Medicine. Available at: https://www.med.nyu.edu/school/md-admissions/mmi-faqs. Accessed May 4, 2015.
[6] Michigan State University College of Human Medicine. Available at: http://mdadmissions.msu.edu/applicants/mmi_faq.php. Accessed May 4, 2015.
[7] University of Arizona College of Medicine. Available at: http://medicine.arizona.edu/admissions/application-process/interviews. Accessed May 4, 2015.
[8] University of Cincinnati College of Medicine. Available at: https://med.uc.edu/medicalstudentadmissions/apply/MMI. Accessed May 4, 2015.
[9] University of Nevada School of Medicine. Available at: http://medicine.nevada.edu/asa/admissions/applicants/selection-factors/applicant-interviews. Accessed May 4, 2015.
[10] University of Saskatchewan. Available at: http://usaskmedalumni.com/2014/09/04/help-our-admissions-office-develop-scenarios-for-testing-students-applying-for-medicine-in-2015/. Accessed May 4, 2015.

Chapter 5

MMI Interviewers

Rule # 9   **Understand who the raters are**

To administer the MMI, the medical school must have one or more raters at each of 8 to 10 stations. A sufficient number of raters must be available for multiple interview dates. Therefore, schools generally train a large number of raters to accommodate their needs. Within several years of instituting the MMI process, Stanford University had recruited 250 raters.[1]

As you would expect, raters are often faculty physicians but the group tends to be heterogeneous at most schools. MMI raters at Stanford University and UC Davis are also lawyers, nurses, former patients, administrators, and residents.

At the McMaster University Michael G. DeGroote School of Medicine in Hamilton, Ontario where the MMI was developed, raters also include students and community members. These have included the former mayor of Hamilton and a copy editor for the *Hamilton Spectator*, Ross Longbottom. Having a variety of stakeholders involved allows the group to bring different perspectives to the interview process. "I take it very seriously," says Mr. Longbottom. "You are actually getting to choose someone who could be standing over you with a scalpel one day."[2]

Unlike the traditional interview where names of interviewers are disclosed to applicants on the interview day, you won't know who your MMI interviewers or raters are until you enter the room to address the MMI question, scenario, or task. Even then, interviewers are often instructed to not indicate their title or position in the medical school. Irrespective of whether your interviewer is a faculty member, student, or community member, rest assured that each rater has been trained to deliver similar interview experiences to every applicant.

Admissions Officers Speak...

"Interviewers are NYU faculty, staff, and students who have been trained specifically for the MMI process at NYU School of Medicine."[3]

New York University School of Medicine

———————

"Interviewers and raters are administrators, faculty, staff, and students who have been trained specifically for the MMI process at the College of Human Medicine. You will not know in what capacity each interviewer/rater is affiliated with the College."[4]

Michigan State University College of Human Medicine

———————

"The 'raters' are actually the individuals who will be positioned at the individual stations. With the MMI process, they are referred to as 'raters' rather than 'interviewers.' The raters are members of the School of Medicine Admissions Committee which includes administrators, faculty, staff, and students and have been trained specifically for the MMI process at Duke."[5]

Duke University School of Medicine

———————

"These people are alumni and community physicians, and members of the larger health care community including nurses, social workers, child health workers, department managers, as well as OHSU faculty, residents and fellows, and students. We have a pool of about 100 that we draw upon..."[6]

Dean Cynthia Morris (Oregon Health & Science University)

Did you know...

During a recent application cycle, the Virginia Tech Carilion School of Medicine received 2,700 applications. From this pool of applicants, 239 were invited to participate in the MMI. Interviews took place over six weekends. The medical school had trained 80 people to serve as interviewers, including doctors and businesspeople from the community.[7]

Rule # 10   Recognize how raters will interact with you.

The way in which interviewers interact with you will differ based on the station type. In a question-based station, you will be given the freedom to address the issue as you see fit. Upon entering the room, you will begin the discussion. At the end of your response, one of two things will happen:

- The interviewer will ask you follow-up questions or;
- The interviewer will inform you that he has all the necessary information.

If the latter occurs before time has run out, you may have to remain in the room until the bell rings.

In a scenario-based station, you will interact with an actor while the interviewer evaluates your performance. The interviewer will function as an observer, and your focus should be entirely on the actor. Don't be surprised or offended if the interviewer doesn't speak or interact with you. It's his or her role to observe.

In a task-based station, you may be paired with another applicant, and the two of you will be assigned a task. As with the scenario-based station, the interviewer will observe your interactions with the other applicant, and rate you accordingly.

Did you know...

During your MMI, your interviewer may ask you probing questions. Some applicants have been unnerved by the aggressiveness of these follow-up questions. Remember that schools may purposely instruct their interviewers to aggressively ask questions as a means to assess your composure and ability to adapt and think quickly on your feet. In some respects, this is similar to the stress interviews that more commonly took place years ago. The advice offered by Dr. Steven Hausrath, a former member of the admissions committee at the University of Texas Medical Branch at Galveston, for stress interviews is certainly applicable to the MMI:[8]

These are stress interviews – we're taught how to give an interview to put some people under stress. Why is that? Because how one reacts to stress is very stereotyped. One reacts to stress in the same way whether it's traffic, a money problem, or whether it's a dilemma at work or in the laboratory. So by provoking a stress response in someone, you get a sense of how they're going to approach a problem or a hurdle. If they become unglued, then that's not a good thing.

Rule # 11   Beware of assessor fatigue.

Even in the MMI, it's common for schools to incorporate questions typically asked during traditional interviews at one or two stations. For example, you may be asked, "Why do you want to be a doctor?" or "Why are you interested in our medical school? In preparing for such questions, work hard to develop answers that would make you stand out from other applicants. This would be of importance even in a traditional interview but MMIs require interviewers to interact with many more applicants. At schools with traditional interviews, the interviewer may have only 3-4 interviews on any given day. Contrast this with the MMI where the interviewer may have to ask the same question to 20 applicants in a short period of time.

As you might expect, interviewers may quickly tire of hearing the same type of answer again and again. This has been termed "assessor fatigue," and has been reported as a concern by MMI interviewers. In one study, researchers described concerns raised by interviewers tasked with asking applicants traditional interview questions. Some representative comments include:

- "It is an essential station, however, after 40 candidates I found it a little tedious."
- "It does allow the prospective student to merely quote prepared answers, often (as many were so similar) written by careers school staff."[9]

Did you know...

In a KevinMD article, I wrote about how applicants often sound the same. Here's an excerpt:[10]

"After a month of interviews, applicants start to blend together. Actually, this starts to happen after a day of interviews. You may provide heartfelt responses, but if you sound like every other applicant, you've lost an important opportunity to stand out and impress. My mantra is: 'If you can imagine another applicant saying the same thing, then your answer isn't good enough.' At a recent symposium, I asked over 300 students to write down their response to this question: 'What are your strengths?' Here are typical answers:

'I am very team oriented and work well with others. I am a calm person who can work well with obstacles that come up, and I am a good listener.'

'My strengths are working well with others, strong listening skills, and work ethic.'

'I have a positive attitude, and constant willingness to learn. I'm easy to work with.'"

> **Did you know...**
>
> Interviewees have been known to ask interviewers for feedback on their performance following their answer. Don't be one of these applicants. Asking for feedback is a huge no-no.

References

[1]Stanford Medicine. Available at: http://med.stanford.edu/news/all-news/2011/11/5-questions-prober-on-new-approach-to-admission-interviews.html. Accessed May 4, 2015.

[2]Globe and Mail. Available at: http://www.theglobeandmail.com/life/interview-20-theres-no-easy-way-to-ace-this-one/article1344084/. Accessed May 4, 2015.

[3]New York University School of Medicine. Available at: https://www.med.nyu.edu/school/md-admissions/mmi-faqs. Accessed May 4, 2015.

[4]Michigan State University College of Human Medicine. Available at: http://mdadmissions.msu.edu/applicants/mmi_faq.php. Accessed May 4, 2015.

[5]Duke University School of Medicine. Available at: http://dukemed.duke.edu/modules/ooa_applicant/index.php?id=9. Accessed May 4, 2015.

[6]Oregon Health & Science University. Available at: http://www.ohsu.edu/xd/education/schools/school-of-medicine/about/school-of-medicine-news/education-news/qa-cynthia-morris.cfm. Accessed June 1, 2015.

[7]New York Times. Available at: http://www.nytimes.com/2011/07/11/health/policy/11docs.html?_r=0. Accessed May 4, 2015.

[8]SUNY Plattsburgh. Available at: http://www.plattsburgh.edu/academics/prehealthadvising/insiderhausrath.php. Accessed May 5, 2015.

[9]McAndrew R, Ellis J. An evaluation of the multiple mini-interview as a selection tool for dental students. *Br Dent J* 2012; 212 (7): 331-5.

[10]KevinMD. Available at: http://www.kevinmd.com/blog/2013/07/medical-school-interview-strategies-admissions-officer.html. Accessed May 3, 2015.

Chapter 6

MMI Experiences of
Prior Interviewees

Rule # 12   **Most interviewees like the MMI. Take comfort in that.**

Multiple studies have shown that most interviewees view the MMI favorably. In a study of 100 applicants who interviewed at the McGill University Faculty of Medicine, researchers found that participants rated the MMI more highly than the traditional interview.[1] Applicants felt that it was fair and enjoyable. Similar results were found in a study of dental students in the United Kingdom with 65% indicating that the MMI was better than the traditional interview.[2]

Medical School Applicants Speak...

"I loved the fact that the MMIs tested to see the type of person you were. The interview process definitely illuminated different characteristics that were necessary for working in the medical field. The different prompts that were given were meant to display your problem-solving abilities, your public health approach, as well as testing your ethics. I feel that having those qualities are crucial to becoming a good physician because it gives you a more holistic view of the patient."[3]

Amy Merino

Did you know...

In a study performed at Chicago Medical School, the MMI was viewed by applicants as a positive interview experience. One hundred percent of the interviewees enjoyed their time on the campus, and the school received positive comments about the MMI.[4]

Medical School Applicants Speak...

"I thought the whole process was more geared toward problem-solving than to me talking about who I was as an applicant. And I liked that."[5]

Andrew Snyder

"You're asked to discuss a given scenario with your interviewer, which I thought was a comparatively objective way to evaluate applicants. Although the combined time is similar to that of the combined time of interviews at other schools, it's a bit more draining since you're constantly being confronted with a new scenario and new interviewer."[6]

Hilary Lin

"Every situation they gave you was very different, including the personal and the ethical. It was better at getting who you are as a person than at other schools. It's part of the reason I picked Robert Wood Johnson."[7]

Bridget Hottenstein

"The scenarios help provide more of a conversation rather than the awkward question-and-short answer situations I found myself in during other interviews. And having multiple interviewers is another aspect of the MMI that I preferred. Each faculty member's impression is considered. I found the MMI to be much less subjective than a single interviewer, who may not consider a student after one wrong answer."[8]

Cory Banaschak

"Prior to my interviewing at Marian, I had experienced a panel interview as well as longer one-on-one interviews. Those interviews were intimidating and felt very formal...it was refreshing to be presented with multiple opportunities to share my interests, my values and my experiences in a unique format. And I felt more at ease knowing that if one station didn't go as well as I had hoped, I still had several others I could excel at."[8]

Heather Chouteau

Rule # 13   **Some applicants are not fans of the MMI. Understand why.**

Although multiple studies have shown that most interviewees view the MMI favorably, a significant percentage of students have expressed concerns. In a study of interviewees at Cardiff University, 10% of participants rated the MMI worse than the traditional interview.[2] As part of this study, qualitative analysis of written comments was performed, and comments were categorized in several themes. Problems cited by interviewees included lack of control, anxiety, and nervousness.

Concerns of Interviewees Following MMI[2]	
Candidate Concern	**Representative Comments**
Lack of control	"…didn't get chance to talk about stuff I wanted to – work experience, personal interests, etc."
	"I felt like it was difficult to express myself at times and put forward my strongest qualities."
	"…five minutes was not enough to fully complete what I had to say."
Anxiety and nervousness	"I was very nervous and did not communicate my thoughts as effectively as I could have."
	"Not calm enough to logically answer the tasks."
Inability to move past poor performance on previous station	"…if the previous station was bad I was nervous for the next one."
Approach taken by interviewers	"Some interviewers were quite aggressive."
McAndrew R, Ellis J. An evaluation of the multiple mini-interview as a selection tool for dental students. *Br Dent J* 2012; 212 (7): 331-5.	

Another concern has to do with the relationship between personality type and MMI scores. In a study performed at UC Davis, researchers had nearly 450 applicants who participated in the MMI process complete a questionnaire. The questionnaire was designed to measure agreeableness, conscientiousness, extroversion, neuroticism, and openness. Of these personality types, conscientiousness had previously been shown to be the personality factor predictive of better performance as a medical student and physician. However, in the study, conscientiousness was not associated with better MMI scores. Instead, researchers found that candidates with higher extroversion scores performed better during the MMI.[9]

Did you know...

In one study, concerns and comments were obtained from MMI interviewers and interviewees during focus group sessions. Some interviewers reported "responding more to the candidates who were confident." This raised concerns among both groups that "students who are more nervous...a little bit shyer" or "less empathic" may be "negatively discriminated against."[10]

Did you know...

In one study, 33% of interviewees considered the MMI to be more stressful than the traditional interview.[11]

Rule # 14   Practice--but be careful not to offer rehearsed answers.

In preparing for the MMI, we do recommend that you read different scenarios and practice by developing responses to these situations. However, some applicants have run into trouble when they offer a rehearsed answer as the response to a similar but not identical scenario. The key is to utilize the knowledge you have gained through preparation, and apply it to the scenario at hand. This will yield a more spontaneous response, and one that will make sense to the interviewer.

Admissions Officers Speak...

"Take time to think about the scenario. Sometimes candidates over-rehearse and don't listen. They answer the question that they've prepared for, rather than responding to what we've said. Quite a few candidates fall down on that."[12]

Micki Regan, Admissions Officer at St. Georges University of London

---

Did you know...

A particularly nice touch is to incorporate information from your background into your answers. For example, if the interviewer asks you about euthanasia and you spent a summer studying the ethics of euthanasia in the Netherlands, work that into your answer. Keep in mind that this is not necessary and you shouldn't overthink this.

References

[1]Razack S, Faremo S, Drolet F, Snell L, Wiseman J, Pickering J. Multiple mini-interviews versus traditional interviews: stakeholder acceptability comparison. *Med Educ* 2009; 43 (10): 993-1000.

[2]McAndrew R, Ellis J. An evaluation of the multiple mini-interview as a selection tool for dental students. *Br Dent J* 2012; 212 (7): 331-5.

[3]Umass Med Now. Available at: http://www.umassmed.edu/news/news-archives/2013/07/mmi-gives-students-multiple-opportunities-to-shine/. Accessed May 4, 2015.

[4]Rosalind Franklin University of Health and Science. Available at: http://www.rosalindfranklin.edu/Portals/0/Documents/Faculty%20Affairs/Faculty%20Development/ERSIG/MMI-ERSIG.pdf. Accessed May 4, 2015.

[5]New York Times. Available at: http://www.nytimes.com/2011/07/11/health/policy/11docs.html?_r=0. Accessed May 4, 2015.

[6]The Stanford Daily. Available at: http://www.stanforddaily.com/2011/07/21/med-school-adopts-multiple-mini-interview-process/. Accessed May 4, 2015.

[7]NJ.com. Available at: http://www.nj.com/news/index.ssf/2011/08/new_interview_process_for_umdn.html. Accessed May 4, 2015.

[8]The DO. Available at: http://thedo.osteopathic.org/2014/09/multple-mini-interviews-gains-traction-schools/. Accessed May 4, 2015.

[9]Jerant A, Griffin E, Rainwater J, Henderson M, Sousa F, Bertakis K, Fenton J, Franks P. Does applicant personality influence multiple mini-interview performance and medical school acceptance offers? *Acad Med* 2012; 87: 1250-59.

[10]Kelly M, Dowell J, Husbands A, Newell J, O'Flynn S, Kropmans T, Dunne F, Murphy A. The fairness, predictive validity and acceptability of multiple mini interview in an internationally diverse student population-a mixed methods study. *BMC Med Educ* 2014; 14: 267.

[11]Dowell J, Lynch B, Till H, Kumwenda B, Husbands A. The multiple mini-interview in the U.K. context: 3 years of experience at Dundee. *Med Teach* 2012; 34 (4): 297-304.

[12]The Guardian. Available at: http://www.theguardian.com/education/2013/oct/07/interview-for-medical-school. Accessed May 4, 2015.

Evaluating Your Performance

Rule # 15   **Understand how the interviewer will evaluate your MMI performance.**

The MMI was pioneered by researchers at the Michael G. DeGroote School of Medicine of McMaster University. University officials have visited institutions across the world offering guidance to medical schools seeking to implement the MMI approach in their own admissions process. To facilitate this process, McMaster University has made several documents public. In the publication *Manual for Interviewers*, you can view the evaluation form used by MMI interviewers at McMaster University.[1] On this form, you will see that the interviewer is asked to rate the applicant's overall performance on a scale of 1 (unsuitable) to 10 (outstanding) relative to the pool of all applicants. The school urges interviewers to carefully consider the following in determining the interview score:

- Communication skills
- Strengths of arguments displayed
- Applicant's suitability for the medical profession

At the bottom of the form is space for the interviewer's comments. Although each school will have its own evaluation form, these criteria will be important to all schools.

Did you know...

"After each six-minute interview is complete, the interviewer gives the candidate a score from one to ten and writes comments on his or her performance. Later, when the executive admissions committee reviews the candidate's full application, they'll be able to see both a composite score and the individual comments and scores from all eight interviewers the candidate met with during his or her MMI session."[2]

New York Medical College

Rule # 16   **Medical schools consider communication to be a vital skill, and will evaluate your proficiency during the MMI.**

"We are trying to weed out the students who look great on paper but haven't developed the people or communication skills we think are important," said Dr. Stephen Workman, Associate Dean for Admissions at the Carilion School of Medicine at Virginia Tech University. "Candidates who jump to improper conclusions, fail to listen or are overly opinionated fare poorly because such behavior undermines teams. Those who respond appropriately to the emotional tenor of the interviewer or ask for more information do well in the new admissions process because such tendencies are helpful, not only with colleagues but also with patients."[3]

If you think about your encounters with doctors, either as a patient or through shadowing, you know that the basis of every physician – patient encounter is a symptom or concern.

To establish the diagnosis, the physician must start by listening carefully and effectively to the patient's story. He then has to ask insightful questions to elicit key information. He must be able to explain even complex diagnoses in terms that are easily understood by the patient. He also has to communicate a treatment plan, and he has to ensure that patient understands and is able to comply with the recommendations.

"Communication skills are important, not only for physicians in their consultations with patients and their families, but also in their contacts with all members of the health care team," writes Dr. Carol Elam, Associate Dean for Admissions at the University of Kentucky College of Medicine.[4]

Given the importance of communication skills in the practice of medicine, medical schools routinely assess for these skills in the admissions interview. In a recent survey of admissions officers, oral communication was assessed at the time of the interview by 91% of schools.[5]

In assessing your communication skills, interviewers seek to answer some very important questions. Are you a good listener? How well do you express yourself? Can you easily engage in conversation? Do you connect with people? The answers to these questions help the interviewer answer the most important question of all: If I were a patient, how would I feel if this person in front of me was my doctor?

Did you know...

Research indicates that patient satisfaction is closely linked to communication behaviors demonstrated by the physician during the physician – patient encounter. Behaviors associated with satisfaction include active listening, responding empathically, and showing concern. Nonverbal communication behaviors shown to be strongly associated with satisfaction include eye contact and listening attentively.

Common Communication Problems Encountered During the MMI

Poor listening skills

In mock and real interviews with med school applicants, I frequently encounter poor listening skills. At question-based stations, after you deliver your initial response, the interviewer will often ask follow-up questions. These may be prompts designed to lead you in a particular direction, and it's up to you to listen carefully to these cues. You may be given new information, and your ability to respond appropriately will yield you extra points. Be sure that you understand the new information. Don't be afraid to ask for clarification if necessary.

Poor nonverbal communication

Don't forget that you'll be communicating in two ways at each station – verbally and nonverbally. Your interviewer will pay close attention to not only what you say but also how you say it. To make a strong favorable impression on your interviewer, be sure to maintain eye contact, display good posture, and avoid distracting behaviors. As obvious as this may seem, I can't tell you how often I encounter applicants who make poor eye contact, slouch in their seats, play with their hair, and fiddle with their pens. Remember that nonverbal communication is important in the physician – patient encounter. Research on the nonverbal behavior of physicians has shown that a comfortable degree of eye contact, head nodding, forward lean, and more direct body orientation with uncrossed arms and legs is viewed positively by patients.

Failure to acknowledge and respond to emotions

In scenario-based stations, there will be times when the actor shows emotion. Many interviewees fail to acknowledge and respond to these emotions. Failure to do so will definitely affect your interview score. Why? Many physicians aren't comfortable with patient emotions, and some even demonstrate blocking behaviors. These include switching topics, ignoring the expressed emotion to focus solely on the physical aspects of the illness, and explaining away distress as normal. If a patient expresses an emotion, it should be acknowledged and further explored. If you put yourself in your patient's shoes, you can imagine how you would feel if your doctor ignored or minimized your fear, sadness, frustration, or anger.

Rule # 17   **You will be told that there are no right or wrong answers. Don't believe that for a minute.**

"There are no right or wrong answers, but instead the MMI gives insight into critical thinking, communication, and decision-making skills."[6]

-    Robin Lorenz, M.D., Ph.D., MSTP Director, University of Alabama at Birmingham

"Oftentimes there are no right or wrong answers to the scenarios posed…"[7]

-    New York University School of Medicine

"There are no right or wrong answers. Instead, the MMI's purpose is to give insight on the applicant's thought process and interpersonal skills as well as individual values and ideals – qualities beyond grades and scores."[8]

-    Michigan State University College of Human Medicine

Is it true? Are there really no right or wrong answers? As reassuring as that sounds, there are clearly wrong answers, and these answers, for the most part, have to do with professionalism. What is professionalism? The foundation of the medical profession rests upon the trust that patients place in their physicians. Professionalism focuses on this foundation of trust. Although it's been defined in many ways, the core values and elements agreed upon include honesty, integrity, compassion, empathy, the ability to communicate effectively with patients, and respect for others.

    Although we think of physicians as highly compassionate and ethical individuals, lapses in ethics and professionalism can affect every level of our profession. These lapses can certainly occur in med school. The evidence indicates that unprofessional behavior in medical school is associated with subsequent disciplinary action of physicians by state medical boards.

In the pressure-packed, high-stakes environment of the MMI, behaviors and attitudes easily surface, particularly when applicants are challenged by interviewers. Your suitability for a career as a physician will be called into question if you:

- Share a belief considered to be unsuitable for a physician. These include, but are not limited to, prejudicial, sexist, or racist comments, statements, or views.

- Choose a position or take a stance that would be considered unethical, highly inappropriate, or immoral for a physician.

- Fail to demonstrate empathy during scenario or task-based encounters with actors or other applicants.

- Lie or cheat

Other ethically inappropriate behaviors and attitudes are presented in the following table.

Ethically Inappropriate Medical Student Behaviors And Attitudes[9]	
Arrogant	Insensitive
Brash	No give and take
Antisocial	Defensive
Rude	Indifferent
Condescending	Prejudiced
Power-seeking	Self-centered
Egocentric	Cocky
Amoral	Dishonest
Rigid attitudes	Selfish
Inflexible	Flippant
Isolated	Uncaring
Devious	Judgmental

It's not always professionalism that calls into question an applicant's suitability for a career in medicine. Responses that convey a lack of understanding about the medical profession or commitment to the field are also concerning to interviewers.

Did you know...

"The system is designed to address the most frequent issue regarding patient complaints. When a licensing or regulatory body reviews the performance of a physician subsequent to patient complaints, the most frequent issues of concern are those of the non-cognitive skills, such as interpersonal skills, professionalism and ethical/moral judgment...The interviewer receives background information on the question or scenario, which assists them in challenging the applicant's ideas or positions. A successful applicant will therefore be one who has used their own body of knowledge effectively and demonstrated a high degree of professionalism in addressing the presented scenario and can deal with the challenges from the interviewer or situation as it develops."[10]

Academy of Medicine

Admissions Officers Speak...

"As a MMI grader, I've seen a couple of people who did pretty bad. One that I interviewed was so nervous she didn't really answer the question. She kept on asking me to give her a minute to think about what she wanted to answer. The other one that stood out the most to me was a girl with that death stare. It's that look when you get into trouble with your significant other but she won't say anything but you know he/she is super pissed."[11]

MMI Interviewer (Student Doctor Network)

Success Tip

In interacting with MMI interviewers at meetings and conferences, I have found that lying or bluffing is particularly concerning. If you encounter a question or scenario that you don't understand, it's always best to ask for clarification.

Did you know...

MMI interviewers have space on the evaluation form to add comments. This space may be used to address concerns about an applicant. In a study done at one school, researchers wrote that "if candidates made one or more inappropriate remarks during the course of any of the station interviews then a 'red flag' option could be employed, indicating that the interviewer had very serious concerns regarding the candidate's suitability for the course and profession."[12]

Rule # 18   **The MMI reduces bias in the interview process but doesn't eliminate it.**

Unlike the traditional interview where the interviewer has access to all or part of your application, MMI interviewers have no knowledge of you as an applicant, including your credentials, background, and accomplishments. "The raters do not know the candidates at all, they have not seen their files, they do not know which undergraduate school they went to, they don't know anything other than their name, and that's because the candidate's wearing a name tag," said Dr. Charles Prober, Associate Dean for Education at Stanford University School of Medicine. "We don't want any bias whatsoever to be introduced into the process."[13]

With no prior knowledge of your background, concerns about introducing bias are lessened. However, bias still remains an issue. Potential sources of bias are described in the following table.

Potential Biases of the Multiple Mini-Interview	
Bias	**Description**
Hawk/dove effect	The evaluator is extremely harsh ("hawk") or lenient ("dove") in his assessment regardless of performance.
Halo effect	The applicant is rated higher across the board because the interviewer permits one factor to overshadow or have an effect on everything else.
Horn effect	The applicant is rated lower across the board because of one factor that is particularly bothersome to the evaluator.
Order effect	Order of interviewees affects evaluation of performance (e.g., scoring an applicant lower or higher because he was interviewed earlier or later among a group of candidates)

Medical school admissions committees work hard to mitigate the effects of any potential bias by training MMI interviewers. As an interviewee, there is little that you can do with respect to the above biases. You can do even less about unconscious biases that some interviewers may have due to stereotypes about race, gender, national origin, sexuality, and disability.

One potential bias deserves further mention because applicants actually have some control over it. This bias has to do with the power of first impressions. We've all heard about the importance of the first impression in making hiring decisions outside of medicine. Is there any evidence to suggest that first impressions are also crucial in medical school interviews? In an interesting study, University of Kentucky anesthesiology residency interviewers made note of their overall impression of applicants within 30 seconds of meeting them, and then determined if these snap judgments correlated with final overall faculty interview scores.[14] A good correlation was indeed found. Although this study was not performed for medical school admissions, residency interviewers often serve on medical school admissions committees. It wouldn't be a stretch to believe that they would be influenced similarly by first impressions when interviewing medical school applicants.

Why do some people make a better first impression than others? "I think a lot of it is a person's interpersonal communications, how they come across," said Dr. Fragneto, lead author of the study. "Do they look you in the eye when they come in? Do they have a firm handshake? Things like that."[14] In my experience conducting mock interviews with medical school applicants, I find that applicants focus almost exclusively on developing answers to questions. Few applicants give considerable thought to the opening of an interview. Since we rarely receive feedback about the first impression we make on others, practice the opening of your interview through role play with others.

Did you know...

The snap judgment an interviewer makes based on their first impression of you can significantly affect your interview score in a positive or negative manner. Your eye contact, posture, smile, attire, and handshake are major determinants of the first impression you will make on the interviewer.

Did you know...

Dr. Charles Prober, Senior Associate Dean for Medical Education, offered some insight into how the medical school reduces interviewer bias in the MMI process. "The structure of MMI mitigates any effect of 'tough scorers' or, at the other extreme, 'rosy-eyed scorers...Because raters see at least eight students on each recruitment day, they serve as their own controls. That is, those raters regarded as being 'tough' are 'tough' for all applicants they see in a given day and their scores are all corrected for their 'toughness.' And because the overall score of each applicant is derived from the score of all eight raters, the effect of a single rater is diluted. Finally, because raters are not given the applicants' files, they are blinded to all prior history and accomplishments and therefore not susceptible to the biases that may arise from a file review."[13]

Rule # 19   Be reassured by the fact that one bad performance will not destroy your chances.

In a traditional medical school interview, the applicant typically has several one-on-one interviews with members of the admissions committee. Each interview is immensely important, and one bad interview can torpedo an applicant's chances of admission. Each MMI interview is also important - but the applicant is exposed to 8 to 10 interviewers, and the opportunity to be evaluated by multiple raters offers applicants an advantage. "Students like the MMI because they have multiple opportunities to shine," said Dr. Mariann Manno, Interim Associate Dean for Admissions at the University of Massachusetts School of Medicine. "With the traditional interview process, a terrific student could have a bad interview. With the MMI, a single bad review can be neutralized by the reviews by multiple other raters."[15]

Success Tip

You must understand that poor performance at a single MMI station can be overcome - but only if you're readily able to move past it. Interviewees who dwell on their suboptimal performance often perform poorly on subsequent stations. This is an incredibly important point, and your ability to embrace and internalize this advice can help you deliver a winning performance.

Medical School Applicants Speak...

"While at first the new MMI format can seem longer and more grueling than the typical interview day, it's important to remember that more interviews means more opportunities to display your personality and interact with representatives from Duke Med. More interviews also means that making one or two mistakes has less of an impact in the overall process."[16]

Hannibal Person, MSIII

Success Tip

Panic is an interviewee's biggest enemy. Nervousness is to be expected, but anxiety and panic can cause well-qualified applicants to act or behave uncharacteristically. Controlling your nerves will allow you to process scenarios and tasks more clearly, and deliver concise and insightful answers that interviewers will find compelling.

Rule # 20   **Show interviewers the strength of your arguments**

In addition to communication skills, interviewers will evaluate the strength of your responses. To show interviewers the strength of your arguments, you must:

- Establish the focus of the topic. Your ability to grasp the underlying issue is very important.

- Identify your own point of view or position. It's important to take a position on the issue. Without it, your argument or discussion will lack clarity and direction. The position you choose should be consistent with the values and characteristics of physicians.

- Present your point of view as a well-reasoned argument. Use compelling reasons to support what you're saying.

- Show the interviewer that you've considered other points of view, and why some might make an argument for these alternative views.

- Deliver your message in a structured way. A well-reasoned argument will not be viewed as such if it is delivered in a disorganized manner. Aim to present your position in a clear and logical way.

Did you know...

"Articulate your thinking process as it is helpful for the interviewer to hear how you arrived at your conclusion and demonstrate that you fully considered all of the information, stakeholders and implications," writes the University of Toronto.[17]

Did you know...

After you've taken a stance and offered reasons for your position, you may find that your interviewer disagrees with you. Don't be surprised by this. Go into every interview expecting to be challenged. As long as you offer reasons for your point of view, you have shown the strength of your argument.

Did you know...

A study of the MMI process performed at the University of Calgary shed some light on how applicants are assessed. The school asked raters to assess interviewees on 5 criteria using a 10-point scale. These criteria included:

- Ability to understand and address the objectives of the scenario
- Communication skills
- Strength of arguments
- Suitability for a career in medicine
- Overall performance

At each station, applicants could be given a maximum of 50 points.[18]

Did you know...

The evaluation form at one medical school allows the rater to express concerns about an applicant's suitability. After ticking the "red flag" box, the rater must describe the concern. Among the examples were rudeness to the rater or another candidate and bizarre statements or mannerisms "suggesting they are unable to conduct themselves in a professional manner."[19]

References

[1]McMaster University. Available at:
http://fhs.mcmaster.ca/mdprog/documents/InterviewerManualFull2012-
13forWEBSITE.pdf. Accessed May 5, 2015.
[2]New York Medical College. Available at:
http://jenuscher.com/static/media/portfolio/transformingbetter.pdf. Accessed May 5,
2015.
[3]New York Times. Available at:
http://www.nytimes.com/2011/07/11/health/policy/11docs.html?_r=0. Accessed May 4,
2015.
[4]Elam C, Burke M, Wiggs J, Speck D. the medical school admission interview:
perspectives on preparation. *NACADA Journal* 1998; 18 (2): 28-32.
[5]Dunleavy D, Whittaker K. The evolving medical school admissions interview. *AIB*
2011; 11 (7).
[6]UAB School of Medicine. Available at:
http://www.uab.edu/medicine/mstp/images/October_2014.pdf. Accessed May 4, 2015.
[7]New York University School of Medicine. Available at:
https://www.med.nyu.edu/school/md-admissions/mmi-faqs. Accessed May 4, 2015.
[8]Michigan State University College of Human Medicine. Available at:
http://mdadmissions.msu.edu/applicants/mmi_faq.php. Accessed May 4, 2015.
[9]Lowe M, Kerridge I, Bore M, Munro D, Powis D. Is it possible to assess the "ethics" of
medical school applicants? *J Med Ethics* 2001; 27 (6): 404-8.
[10]Academy of Medicine. Available at:
http://www.academyofmedicine.org/Portals/0/MMI%20Description.pdf. Accessed May
4, 2015.
[11]Student Doctor Network. Available at: http://www.studentdoctor.net/. Accessed May 3,
2015.
[12]Perkins A, Burton L, Dray B, Elcock K. Evaluation of a multiple mini-interview
protocol used as a selection tool for entry to an undergraduate nursing program. *Nurse
Educ Today* 2013; 33 (5): 465-9.
[13]The Stanford Daily. Available at: http://www.stanforddaily.com/2011/07/21/med-
school-adopts-multiple-mini-interview-process/. Accessed May 4, 2015.
[14]Anesthesiology News. Available at:
http://www.anesthesiologynews.com/ViewArticle.aspx?d=Ad+Lib&d_id=384&i=Septe
mber2011&i_id=760&a_id=18916. Accessed May 5, 2015.
[15]UMass Med Now. Available at: http://www.umassmed.edu/news/news-
archives/2013/07/mmi-gives-students-multiple-opportunities-to-shine/. Accessed May 4,
2015.
[16]DukeMed. Available at: http://www.dukedavisoncouncil.org/?page_id=258. Accessed
May 5, 2014.
[17]University of Toronto. Available at:
http://www.utsc.utoronto.ca/aacc/sites/utsc.utoronto.ca.aacc/files/u5/PreparingforMMI.pd
f. Accessed May 4, 2015.
[18]Lemay J, Lockyer J, Collin V, Brownell A. Assessment of non-cognitive traits through
the admissions multiple mini-interview. *Med Educ* 2007; 41 (6): 573-79.
[19]Dowell J, Lynch B, Till H, Kumwenda B, Husbands A. The multiple mini-interview in
the U.K. context: 3 years of experience at Dundee. *Med Teach* 2012; 34 (4): 297-304.

Chapter 8

Basics of Preparation

Rule # 21   **Don't buy into the belief that you can't prepare for the MMI.**

You'll hear that it's difficult to prepare for the MMI, and schools may even urge you to not prepare in certain ways. "It is not recommended that you try to prepare for specific MMI questions," writes the University of Nevada School of Medicine.[1] "Reviewing or going through a list of 'practice' questions is not applicable because the MMI does not use the same questions as a standard interview," writes the University of Cincinnati College of Medicine.[2]

The truth is that it's important to prepare because preparation can help you in a variety of ways:

- It takes poise and presence to deliver strong answers to MMI questions, and practicing will help you develop the confidence needed to tackle these challenging situations.

- Moving from one station to another requires you to be flexible and open to encountering new situations, and practicing through a circuit of stations allows you to more easily adapt to MMI questions and scenarios.

- Communication skills will be assessed at each station, and the feedback you receive through practice will leave you better informed about your ability to speak articulately.

- Like other types of medical school admissions interviews, the MMI is a high stakes interview, and applicants will understandably be anxious. Practicing will help you handle your "nerves," and show you how to channel this energy to elevate your performance.

A Few Key Pointers

In the following 5 chapters, we're going to provide further guidance to help you prepare for the different types of MMI prompts. While there's no set of rules that will work for every possible scenario or question you might be faced with, we do recommend keeping a few key pointers in mind. We call these the P6C, and we've focused on these because applicants often make errors related specifically to these 7 areas.

The P6C	
Professional: How would a professional respond?	How would a physician respond to this scenario? In the medical profession, displaying compassion and empathy in all our interactions is critical.
	How would a physician speak? Seek feedback on your verbal communication skills.
	How would a physician walk into the room? Seek feedback on your nonverbal communication skills: your posture, handshake, eye contact, and smile
	See case of freezing eggs from deceased donor
Prompt: Read the prompt. Now reread the prompt.	Many scenarios or questions have extra information or startling details that may distract from the actual prompt.
	Make sure you have identified and verbalized the prompt correctly.
	For example, some prompts specifically ask "what would you do?", while others ask "discuss the issues involved."
	See case on right to die
Priorities: A strong response explicitly states your priorities.	For a medical question, your priority is often (but not always) patient care.
	See case on Ebola virus quarantine.
Perspectives: Consider all perspectives.	Consider all stakeholders when you're formulating a response.
	This may include the perspectives of patients, family members, physicians, nurses, employers, hospitals, insurers, taxpayers, the community, the nation's healthcare system, and others.
	See case on pricing transparency in healthcare

A Few Key Pointers: The P6C	
Probe further: Don't jump to conclusions.	If you're responding to a scenario, never jump to conclusions. It's important to look for other possible explanations.
	If acting, it's important to ask more questions.
	If describing your response to a challenging scenario, it's important to verbalize other possible explanations.
	See case of employee using cell phone at work
Problem-solving: Look for other potential solutions.	In responding to challenging scenarios, it's rare to find a scenario in which there are only two potential solutions.
	Creative problem-solving can usually identify other options.
	See case of patient refusing to wear a mask
Conclusion: End with a strong conclusion	Why does this get its own rule? Because it's such a common mistake.
	Sometimes applicants have a hard time wrapping up their thought processes.
	It's important to end on a strong note and leave a strong final impression.
	Make sure you conclude with a strong summary sentence, leaving time for follow-up questions.

Admissions Officers Speak...

"Because you will be rotating through several different stations and because the MMI does not use the same questions you might experience during a traditional interview, we do not recommend that you attempt to rehearse answers ahead of time. Instead, we recommend you practice expressing yourself verbally to someone else to ensure that you can provide thorough, logical answers within a short time frame."[3]

New York University School of Medicine

"As with any human interaction, practice is helpful. It could identify nervous habits, and it may help you feel more comfortable and relaxed. Participate in a mock interview event through your school's career development office, have a friend ask questions and give you feedback, or use a webcam to record your own practice responses. All of these may help you find ways in which you might improve your interview performance."[4]

Michigan State University College of Human Medicine

"The strongest advice is to understand the basic structure, time limit, and number of stations. Listen carefully to any prompts directed to you."[5]

Duke University School of Medicine

"The purpose of the MMI is not to test your scientific or clinical knowledge. However, you may find it helpful to be familiar with current events and policies in health care."[6]

University of Arizona College of Medicine

"Your time is best spent learning how to discuss your thoughts and ideas in a brief timeframe so you can provide the most logical and thorough answers at each station. Recording your answers can help you improve your performance."[1]

University of Nevada School of Medicine

Rule # 22   **Become knowledgeable about current events, ethical issues, and social policies.**

"We recognized that our biggest problem is not in evaluating the cognitive domain - it's not about knowledge," says Dr. Jack Rosenfeld, Professor Emeritus of Pathology and Molecular Medicine and Co-Creator of the MMI. "It's the interpersonal domain: the way of dealing with people. It's about ethics and it's about judgment."[7] You will hear that MMI stations are not designed to be a test of your scientific or pre-existing medical knowledge, and that is true. However, some stations have a medical aspect, often dealing with current events, ethical issues, or social policies. Ethical issues are particularly common.

What are your thoughts about the role of the pharmaceutical industry in medical practice? How would you handle a case of witnessed medical negligence by a colleague? Have you thought about the ethics of end-of-life care?

You need to.

You must be prepared to respond to ethical dilemmas during an interview. In an analysis of interviewee experiences, researchers found that approximately 10% of interview questions focused on resolving an ethical dilemma. The authors wrote that "admissions committees and faculty physicians deem it important to query prospective students about ethical issues."[8]

"Controversial and ethical topics have become somewhat standard among medical school interviews. They are worth researching in advance, and thus a word to the wise is: DO YOUR HOMEWORK."[9]

> Dr. Norma Wagoner
> Former Dean of Students
> University of Chicago Pritzker School of Medicine

Interviewers may present you with a difficult scenario, and ask how you would resolve it. You're more likely to respond well if you have a basic understanding of the issues surrounding the dilemma. You'll need to become well-read on common controversies in medicine.

Since it's not possible to prepare for every possible scenario, we recommend that when you're faced with questions about a difficult and complex ethical situation you:

- Pause to gather your thoughts. What do you know of the situation based on your experiences and reading?

- Ask for clarification or further information, if needed.

- Share your knowledge of the topic with the interviewer.

- Discuss, out loud, the steps you would take to resolve the situation so the interviewer can assess your analytical and reasoning skills.

- Provide an answer or present options, and explain your rationale.

You won't simply be judged on the content of your answer. Questions about ethical scenarios are used to assess your poise under stress. Interviewers also assess your ability to "think on your feet," and they'll evaluate your approach to a difficult situation. Do you ask for more information if you feel that something is missing? Are you open to seeking input from others?

You should avoid being "quick to judge, quick to respond without gathering data, or imposing your opinion on the patient when your opinions differ," writes Dr. Carol Teitz, Associate Dean for Admissions at the University of Washington School of Medicine. Dr. Teitz finds it acceptable to say, "I don't know," but this should be followed with "Here's how I would go about making a decision."[10]

How will your response to an ethical issue be evaluated?

Interviewers will look to answer the following questions in assessing your response:

- Did the interviewee identify the specific ethical issues or problems?

- Was the interviewee able to analyze the issues?

- What was the strength of the argument?

- Did the interviewee consider other viewpoints or perspectives?

- How well did the interviewee express his ideas or thoughts?

- Was the applicant's viewpoint or recommendation suitable and reasonable?

Common Ethical Dilemmas Asked of Medical School Applicants

- Doctor – patient relationship

- Confidentiality
- Informed consent
- Patient rights
- End-of-life decisions
- Patient autonomy
- Truth telling/disclosure

- Professionalism/professional misconduct

- Medical negligence/mistakes

- Relationship with pharmaceutical industry

- Issues related to reproductive health

- Issues related to treatment of HIV/AIDS

- Genetics/stem cell

- Issues related to treatment of mentally ill patients

- Performing procedures/tests not medically indicated for reasons for defensive medicine

- Disagreements between patients/families and physicians about treatment decisions

- Treatment with placebo

- Transplantation/organ donation

- Research ethics

- Abortion

- Physician-assisted suicide

- Physician impairment (alcohol, drugs, or illness)

- Conflicts of interest

- Health care rationing

- Introducing medical students as doctors

- Practicing procedures on anesthetized or dead patients

Rule # 23   **Practice makes perfect.**

Many applicants have a difficult time discussing issues logically and coherently. In the following box, we've presented some ways for you to improve your skills in this area. Our recommendations begin with becoming more knowledgeable about ethics, current events, social policies, and the health system. With knowledge in hand, you'll be ready to practice expressing your ideas about these issues with others. Your ability to form and verbalize your thoughts will improve. "Practice with someone you don't know, as that'll help you to get used to an interview situation and to role plays," says Kim Piper, Lecturer at Queen Mary University. "Any student who practices questions with an adult they don't know well will find it easier. Doing that can help to get rid of nerves."[11] Utilize the feedback you receive to make your presentations even better.

How should I prepare for the MMI?

- Read about ethics.

- Become well informed about the health system.

- Gather MMI questions and scenarios from the Internet, and practice delivering timed presentations to a partner or friend.

- Pay close attention to the news, and practice debating issues with family and friends.

- Read the Op-Ed section of the newspaper to understand how an argument or persuasive piece is presented.

- Learn from the opinions and viewpoints of others.

- Encourage others to present to you a topic, and then deliver an impromptu discussion.

- Consider taking a public speaking class.

- Join Toastmasters.

- Attend MMI sessions conducted by your premedical advising office.

- View videos of MMI encounters developed by medical schools. These videos are available at school websites and YouTube.

- Record yourself answering questions to assess your verbal and nonverbal communication.

Rule # 24   Respect the power of voice.

You've reviewed the school's mission statement and philosophy. You feel confident about your attire. Your mock interviewer was impressed with the quality of your handshake. You've prepared exhaustively for ethical questions. What have you overlooked? Chances are you haven't given any thought to your voice.

As an exercise, listen to the speaking voices of others in public, particularly people whom you've never met. You'll find that you quickly draw impressions of people based on the quality, volume, pitch, and pace of their speaking voice. In the MMI process, where your encounter with the interviewer will last no longer than 8 minutes, your voice will have considerable impact on the way in which you are perceived. You can say all the right things, but if your voice is not consistent with your message, you'll fail to inspire confidence in the interviewer. As far as voice is concerned, here's what I commonly encounter in mock interviews:

- Weak or timid voice

  Your goal is to project your voice strongly. Unfortunately, the high stakes setting of the interview can easily make your voice sound weak.

- Speaking too loudly

  This tends to be less common in my experience, but could communicate an overbearing or aggressive nature.

- Speaking too fast

  Nervousness and concern about running out of time can cause applicants to speak too quickly. The end result is stumbling over words.

- Trailing off at the end of a response

- Pronouncing statements as if they were questions ("uptalk")

  Uptalk occurs when speakers end their sentences with rising inflection, making it seem as if the statement is a question. Believed to have originated in the Valley Girl culture of California, it was popularized in the movie *Clueless*. Although more common in women, it's not at all unusual in men. In an interesting study, contestants on the game show *Jeopardy!* used uptalk 37% of the time.[12] Unfortunately, in interview settings uptalk has been found to be detrimental.

- Vocal fry

   Vocal fry is different than uptalk, and refers to a low-pitched, creaky-sounding speech inflection. You can easily find examples of vocal fry on YouTube. It's become a common type of speech, and research indicates that women who demonstrate vocal fry come across as less competent.

Did you know...

How important is the sound of your voice? In an analysis of speeches delivered by 120 executives, researchers at Quantified Impressions determined that the sound of a speaker's voice accounted for 23% of listeners' evaluations. Of note, it was rated more important than the content of the message (11%). "We are hard-wired to judge people," says Lynda Stucky, president of ClearlySpeaking. "You hear somebody speak, and the first thing you do is to form an opinion about them."[13]

If you're like most people, you've probably never received any feedback on your voice. In your interview preparation, seek opinions about your voice quality from others. An especially effective but underutilized technique is to videotape your mock interview so that you can hear what you sound like. Was your voice rough or weak? Were you speaking too fast? Don't fret if you discover any problems. Knowing about problems in advance of your interview will allow you to take the steps needed to convey calmness and strength through your voice. Although many applicants assume that nothing can be done to change voice quality, that's not at all true. You can strengthen or improve your voice with coaching.

Did you know...

It can be hard for many applicants to avoid fillers, such as "uh" and "um." With practice, however, you can replace these fillers with brief pauses. Take several seconds to gather your thoughts before you continue. Initially, this pause may seem like an eternity but it won't be perceived as such by the interviewer. Effective utilization of pauses shows confidence and adds variety.

Rule # 25   Ready for questions about health policy? You need to be.

Being asked questions about health policy and politics are among interviewees' worst fears. "These questions can be a minefield of potential admissions-killing errors," says Dr. Nathan Moore, author of *The Health Care Handbook.*[14]

Several years ago, I wrote an article for *PreMedLife* to help medical school interviewees deliver strong responses to health care questions. Below is the article.[15]

How to Nail Interview Questions about Health Care

"Congratulations! After review of your application, our Medical School Admissions Committee would like to invite you for an interview." *These are the words that every medical school applicant hopes to read.*

In an AAMC survey of medical schools, the interview was found to be the most important factor in the admissions process.

To prepare, applicants consider how to respond to anticipated questions. Why do you want to be a doctor? Why are you interested in our school? Why should we choose you? While these questions are challenging, my experience advising applicants has shown us that questions about current healthcare issues provoke the most anxiety.

PREPARE TO BE ASKED QUESTIONS ABOUT CURRENT HEALTHCARE ISSUES

- What can be done about rising health costs?
- How could you affect the health care system?
- How do you see the field of medicine changing in the next ten years?
- What do you think of the government's involvement in health care?
- What is your understanding of the Affordable Care Act?

Prepare to be asked these questions. As medical school admissions interviewers, we ask these questions. We know that our colleagues ask these questions. "I think ALL students applying to medical school should be prepared for questions about the healthcare system and reform," says Dr. Gregory Polites, Associate Professor of Emergency Medicine at the Washington University School of Medicine. "Now more than ever, it's crucial that both students and physicians keep abreast of the changes that are occurring now and will occur in the future."[16]

UNDERSTAND THE IMPORTANCE OF THESE QUESTIONS

A review of medical school websites reveals the importance of these questions in the interview process:

- "Specifically, the interviewers will try to determine…What do you know about the practice of medicine and issues in delivery of health care?"[17] (University of Washington School of Medicine)

- "You may be asked to discuss a controversial issue or situations dealing with ethics or professionalism in health care. Be aware of current issues and recent debates in the health field."[18] (Florida State University College of Medicine)

- Qualities searched for in an interview…Knowledge of health care systems and its current changes."[19] (Texas Tech University School of Medicine)

"Given the critical nature of health care in our country I feel every prospective medical student should have at least a general understanding of the more salient parts of the national health care policy," says Dr. Will Ross, Associate Dean for Diversity at the Washington University School of Medicine. "I expect them to defend their rationale for why health care reform is moving well, flawed, or fine as is. I will then comment in my interview summary on whether the applicant has a pedestrian, mature, or sophisticated understanding of health care reform."[20]

UNDERSTAND WHAT THE INTERVIEWER IS SEEKING

Rest assured that your interviewer does not expect you to be well versed in the nuances of healthcare reform. With that being the case, what is the purpose of these questions?

"This interaction tells the interviewers that the candidate has some awareness of the wider world and that she or he is cognizant of the changes in the health care system that may have complex implications for practitioners," writes Dr. Carol Elam, Associate Dean for Admissions at the University of Kentucky College of Medicine. "Neither is the applicant expected to have extensive knowledge of the subject. Rather, this discussion gives the interviewer a chance to see that the candidate, in preparing for a career in medicine, is aware of the issues confronting the profession."[21]

With the changes that are occurring in our health care system, schools seek to identify students who have an interest in finding solutions to our nation's health care problems. "Just as we learn to diagnose diseases and develop treatment plans for individual patients, we must also learn to diagnose and treat problems in the systems," writes Dr. Paul Rockey, former Associate Dean for Clinical Affairs at the Southern Illinois University School of Medicine. "Too often our profession has left this task to administrators, regulators, and insurers. Medical care doesn't end when we leave the patient's bedside or exit the examining room."[22]

BECOME WELL INFORMED OF HEALTHCARE ISSUES

If you're feeling unprepared to handle these questions, take comfort in knowing that others feel the same. University of Michigan researchers surveyed more than 58,000 graduating U.S. medical students from 2003 – 2007. Nearly half of the students felt inadequately prepared in understanding the health care system, health economics, managed care, or managing a practice.[23] In another survey of over 800 medical students in Minnesota, researchers sought to determine knowledge of the 2010 Affordable Care Act. Less than half reported understanding the law's basic components.[24] To increase knowledge of health care issues, schools have incorporated coursework into their curricula. "Ten or 15 years ago, most schools did not have anything involving health care policy," said Dr. Matthew Mintz, Associate Professor of Medicine at George Washington University in an interview with Slate. "Medicine was medicine and policy was policy and why would doctors want to learn anything about policy?"[25] Today, most medical schools include health policy, business and/or delivery teaching along with traditional subjects like anatomy and pathology.

Medical students have also taken the initiative to develop resources to enhance understanding of complex issues in the health care system. One such text is the *Health Care Handbook* written by Elisabeth Askin and Nathan Moore, students at the Washington University School of Medicine. "We wanted to write a book that would be like giving people little floaties to help them learn to swim through the vast and confusing ocean that is health care," said Elisabeth in an interview with the *New York Times*.[26] Other recommended resources to help you become well informed include American Medical News, AMSA The New Physician, Virtual Mentor, KevinMD, and the New York Times Health Section.

With your interview invitation in hand, you are one step closer to your goal: medical school. Although developing an understanding of the health care system may seem daunting, now is the time to recognize current healthcare issues, identify gaps in your knowledge, and take steps to expand your understanding. It's well worth the effort.

Some Additional Tips On Handling Interview Questions About The Affordable Care Act

- Understand that the Affordable Care Act (ACA) may be an emotionally charged topic for interviewers. Physicians will have varying opinions about the ACA.
- Some physicians are strong proponents of the ACA while others are fierce opponents. A 2015 survey showed that 44% of physicians were opposed to the ACA prior to implementation. The percentage opposed rose to 58% one year after its implementation.[27]
- Therefore, you must be delicate in how you answer questions. Fortunately, you can provide an informed response without indicating a strong political preference. To do so, be sure to include both pros and cons in your answer.
- In the aforementioned survey, positives included increased access to care for patients, coverage for children under 26, reduced costs of end-of-life care, emphasis on preventive medicine, and no insurance denials for pre-existing conditions.
- Negatives included reduced reimbursement to physicians, increased patient debt due to high-deductible plans, and practice burdens related to administrative hassles.
- A particularly useful strategy is to become informed about how the ACA is being implemented in the state in which the medical school you will be visiting is located. You can then utilize this knowledge in your MMI answer.

References

[1]University of Nevada School of Medicine. Available at: http://medicine.nevada.edu/asa/admissions/applicants/selection-factors/applicant-interviews. Accessed May 8, 2015.

[2]University of Cincinnati College of Medicine. Available at: https://med.uc.edu/medicalstudentadmissions/apply/MMI. Accessed May 7, 2015.

[3]New York University School of Medicine. Available at: https://www.med.nyu.edu/school/md-admissions/mmi-faqs. Accessed May 4, 2015.

[4]Michigan State University College of Human Medicine. Available at: http://mdadmissions.msu.edu/applicants/mmi_faq.php. Accessed May 4, 2015.

[5]DukeMed. Available at: http://www.dukedavisoncouncil.org/?page_id=258. Accessed May 5, 2014.

[6]University of Arizona College of Medicine. Available at: http://medicine.arizona.edu/admissions/application-process/interviews. Accessed May 4, 2015.

[7]The Globe and Mail. Available at: http://www.theglobeandmail.com/life/interview-20-theres-no-easy-way-to-ace-this-one/article1344084/. Accessed May 7, 2015.

[8]Rippentrop A, Wong M, Altmaier E. A content analysis of interviewee reports of medical school admissions interviews. Available at: http://www.med-ed-online.org. Accessed May 5, 2015.

[9]Association of American Medical Colleges. Available at: https://www.aamc.org/students/aspiring/basics/284816/interview6.html. Accessed May 5, 2015.

[10]University of Washington School of Medicine. Available at: http://www.uwmedicine.org/education/Documents/md-program/TheInterview%2014.pdf. Accessed May 4, 2015.

[11]The Guardian. Available at: http://www.theguardian.com/education/2013/oct/07/interview-for-medical-school. Accessed May 4, 2015.

[12]Linneman T. Gender in *Jeopardy!* Intonation variation on a television game show. *Gender & Society* 2013; 27 (1): 82-105.

[13]The Wall Street Journal. Available at: http://www.wsj.com/articles/SB10001424127887323735604578440851083674898. Accessed May 5, 2015.

[14]Student Doctor Network. Available at: http://www.studentdoctor.net/2014/12/discussing-obamacare-in-your-med-school-interviews/. Accessed May 22, 2015.

[15]PreMedLife (September/October 2013). Available at: http://www.premedlife.com/feature-articles/how-to-nail-interview-questions-about-health-care-1459/. Accessed May 22, 2015.

[16]Dr. Gregory Polites (personal communication).

[17]University of Washington School of Medicine. Available at: http://www.uwmedicine.org/education/md-program/admissions/applicants/pages/interview.aspx. Accessed June 16, 2013.

[18]Florida State University College of Medicine. Available at: http://med.fsu.edu/?page=mdAdmissions.interview. Accessed June 17, 2013.

[19]Texas Tech University School of Medicine. Available at: http://www.ttuhsc.edu/som/admissions/umsi.aspx. Accessed June 17, 2013.

[20]Dr. Will Ross (personal communication).

[21]Elam C, Burke M, Wiggs J, Speck D. The medical school admission interview: perspectives on preparation. *NACADA Journal* 1998; 18 (2): 28 – 32.

[22]Rockey P, Winship M. Nurturing leaders for an environmental change. Available at: http://virtualmentor.ama-assn.org/2009/11/pfor1-0911.html. Accessed June 15, 2013.

[23]Patel M, Lypson M, Davis M. Medical student perceptions of education in health care systems. *Acad Med* 2009; 84 (9): 1301-6.

[24]Winkelman T, Antiel R, Davey C, Tilburt J, Song J. Medical students and the Affordable Care Act: uninformed and undecided. *Arch Intern Med* 2012; 172 (20): 1603-5.

[25]Beam C. Is our doctors learning? Why aren't medical students taught about health care policy? Available at: http://www.slate.com/articles/news_and_politics/prescriptions/2009/06/is_our_doctors_learning.html. Accessed June 15, 2013.

[26]Chen P. Two medical students navigate the health care maze. Available at: http://well.blogs.nytimes.com/2012/07/12/two-medical-students-navigate-the-health-care-maze/. Accessed June 17, 2013.

[27]LocumTenens.com Survey. Available at: http://www.prnewswire.com/news-releases/66-percent-of-physicians-feel-the-affordable-care-act-should-be-repealed-300044607.html. Accessed May 22, 2015.

Chapter 9

Question/Discussion Station Preparation

In this chapter, I'll present a question/discussion station approach that will significantly increase your chances of making a favorable impression on the interviewer. In later chapters, I'll address approaches for scenario- and task-based stations, followed by an overview of behavioral interview questions. The differences between these types of MMI stations were reviewed in Chapter 4.

Rule # 26   **Set the stage for success by making the most of your first two minutes.**

In the typical MMI format, you'll be presented with a question posted on the door. You'll typically have **two minutes** to read this information and gather your thoughts. An alarm will then ring, signaling that it's time for you to enter the room where you will respond to the question. These can be complex issues to address, and candidates often wonder if it's possible to deliver a cogent response in a time-limited manner. Without a doubt, you can, and making the most of these two minutes will set the stage for a successful encounter.

      In these precious two minutes, I recommend that you begin by focusing on the topic. As obvious as this may seem, in my MMI mock interview sessions, I have seen how easy it is for applicants to squander this time by allowing the mind to wander or become overwhelmed with feelings of nervousness. Begin by determining the focus of the scenario or question. Is it an ethical scenario about confidentiality? Is it a scenario assessing your integrity or professionalism?

> **Did you know...**
>
> "I have been an interviewer during an MMI for a healthcare institution...the best thing I can tell you is *read the question and read it again*. Applicants occasionally came in to my room having not the faintest clue what the parameters were, and came prepared to follow some instructions in their head that were nothing like what they were supposed to be doing. That always left me underwhelmed."[1]

Rule # 27   Define the structure of your response.

Once you've identified the topic, it's time to develop your plan or approach. By defining a structure to what you will say, you'll enter the room with a more organized approach. This will help prevent rambling, one of the most common mistakes interviewees make. The response you give at a question station should include an introduction, body, and conclusion. Think of it as a speech, granted an impromptu one. All good speeches have these three parts. I recommend that you:

- Lead with a compelling introduction.

- Select an appropriate approach for the body of your discussion.

   - Discuss 3-4 important points that come to mind about the topic.

   - Discuss the pros and cons of an issue, or talk about two sides of the issue.

   - State your point of view and give the reason that you feel this way, providing support for your views. Show that you've considered other points of view.

   - Think of the past, present, and future. There was a time when...but now we find that...in the future I expect...

   - Ask yourself who, what, when, where, why and how and focus on the response to those questions in your discussion.

   - Discuss how the topic affects you personally or how it affects the world in general.

- End with a strong conclusion.

Did you know...

On your notepad or card, quickly write down an introduction, two or three supporting points, and a conclusion, or use another approach as shown above. If you're not permitted to use notes, learn how to organize your thoughts in your mind.

Rule # 28   Manners matter

Not long ago, I came across an interesting discussion in an online patient forum. Although contributors to the discussion felt that doctors generally knocked before entering rooms, some were miffed by what sometimes happened next. Rather than waiting for permission to open the door, doctors sometimes just barged right in after knocking. For the busy physician trying desperately to stay on schedule, this breach in door-knocking etiquette may seem trivial. However, it's an important part of the first impression that we make on our patients, and can set the stage for a satisfying and positive physician-patient encounter. Some other reasons why patients appreciate this behavior:

- The patient may not have disrobed or fully changed into the gown.

- The patient may be anxious about the visit. A few seconds may allow the patient to regain composure.

- While waiting, the patient may have chosen to make a phone call or read a book. Waiting for permission to enter the room permits the patient to end a phone conversation or set aside a book.

"Basic etiquette-based communication makes a difference in patient outcomes, but it doesn't appear that these strategies are being used to the extent that they should be," says Dr. Leonard Feldman, Assistant Professor of Medicine at Johns Hopkins University School of Medicine. "These communication strategies matter to patients and are relatively easy to do."[2] As an aspiring physician, you can demonstrate proper etiquette in the MMI, starting with knocking on the door and waiting for permission to enter the room.

> **Did you know…**
>
> "I believe that medical education and postgraduate training should place more emphasis on this aspect of the doctor–patient relationship — what I would call 'etiquette-based medicine.' There have been many attempts to foster empathy, curiosity, and compassion in clinicians, but none that I know of to systematically teach good manners. The very notion of good manners may seem quaint or anachronistic, but it is at the heart of the mission of other service-related professions."[3]
>
> Michael Kahn, M.D.

Rule # 29   Buy yourself some extra time if necessary

"At one MMI station, I got confused about the wording of the question and realized that I read the question wrong 20s after I started to reply. I stumbled around for a bit trying to sneak extended glances at the prompt, so I could figure out what the heck was going on in the scenario! The interviewer had to ask me clarify what I meant a couple of times. By the time I figured it out, time was just about up."[4]

-        Medical School Applicant (Student Doctor Network)

If you find yourself struggling after the two minutes elapse, consider one of the following approaches, assuming that the MMI process at the school permits it:

- Enter the room and ask for clarification if there is something you don't understand.

- Enter the room and ask if you can have a moment before you speak.

- Enter the room and look over the scenario or question again. Often, there will be a second copy of the instructions inside the room.

Although any one of the above approaches will cut into the time you have available to address the issue, the time you've bought may be just what you need to help you gather your thoughts and regain your composure. Although this is a potential strategy, refrain from utilizing it too often. Schools are assessing you on your ability to think on your feet.

Try not to start any discussion with "I'm really not good at this," "I don't know where to begin," or "I don't have a clue how to answer this." These are comments that I've frequently encountered in mock interview situations. Hopefully you'll be able to avoid saying something to this effect if you can buy yourself some additional time.

If you just don't have any experience or knowledge of the topic…

Think about your knowledge or experience in a similar area, and consider offering it instead.

Admit that you don't have the answer but then describe how you would solve the problem. "Although I don't know the answer to the question, I'd like to tell you how I would go about finding the answer…"

Rule # 30   **The power of first impressions and the importance of non-verbal communication.**

Never underestimate the power of the first impression. As soon as you enter the room, pause to introduce yourself (unless you've been given instructions not to do so). Your appearance, attire, smile, posture, eye contact, and handshake are all components of the first impression. We generally make assumptions based on our first impressions, and these are rarely based on feedback. It's wise to practice the opening of an interview with a mock interviewer. This can help you develop an understanding of how you come across when you're meeting someone new. Do you walk with confidence? Are you standing tall? Do you have a nice, engaging smile? Are you making good eye contact?

Did you know…

When meeting someone for the first time, 93% of the first impression you make will be based on nonverbal communication (e.g., body language, attitude, demeanor, etc.). Only 7% of your first impression is based on what you say.

Body Language Tips Following The First Impression

What should I do with my hands?

Rest your hands in your lap. It's acceptable to clasp your hands together, but don't clasp them too tightly or make a fist. Avoid folding your arms across your chest. This can create an impression of rigidity, unapproachability, or even dishonesty. Do not cover your mouth or touch your face while you speak. Avoid touching your tie, tugging at your collar, or straightening your clothing. We also recommend that you not hold your pen in your hand. Many applicants end up fiddling or tapping with it.

How should I sit?

Posture can weigh heavily in how others perceive you. Maintain an alert, straight posture while you sit, stand, and walk. Leaning forward slightly while sitting demonstrates interest but don't lean on the table or desk. Applicants who slouch can appear lazy, unmotivated, or disinterested.

What should I do with my feet?

Keep your feet flat on the floor. You may cross your legs at your ankles. Do not rest your ankle on the opposite knee.

Rule # 31   Start with a strong introduction

Starting with a strong introduction is not as hard as some applicants believe. If you are able to grasp the meaning or significance of the issue, you can certainly craft a strong opening. You can build momentum for the rest of your response with a strong opening. In the event that you lose your train of thought during the discussion, you can return to what you've said in the opening to redirect yourself. Consider the following MMI scenario:

Mr. C, a 72-year old male with mild dementia, diabetes and elevated cholesterol, is admitted to the hospital with right leg pain and swelling following a long plane trip. The emergency medicine physician has made the diagnosis of deep vein thrombosis (DVT), a condition that poses considerable risk to the patient's health. The danger with this condition is that the blood clot that has formed within the veins in the patient's leg could travel to the blood vessels supplying the lungs, causing a potentially life-threatening condition termed pulmonary embolism (PE). The treatment of DVT is the blood thinner heparin. Despite the best efforts of the medical team, the patient is steadfast in his refusal to start heparin or any other blood thinner. He simply states, "If my time has come, then I'm ready to accept it." Unwilling to accept the patient's decision, the intern says, "We need to find a way to force this patient to take this medication." Discuss the ethical issues involved.

A particularly effective technique is to enter the room and summarize the question, issue, or scenario in your own words:

In this particular case, the patient has been diagnosed with a serious condition. He has been found to have a blood clot. If it travels to the lungs, he could become seriously ill or even die. The treatment for the clot is a blood thinner but the patient refuses to take the medication despite the pleas of the medical team. This has frustrated the intern, and he wants to find a way to make the patient take the medication. Do you feel that I have a good understanding of the situation?

Beginning with a summary of the issue is similar to what physicians do during patient encounters. After we take a history, we will often check the accuracy of what we've heard by offering the patient a summary and an opportunity to correct any errors in our history taking. "Let me see if I have this right...Your symptoms started...You first noticed..." You can do the same during the MMI, and it will be viewed favorably.

After checking in with the interviewer to verify your understanding of the issue or question, continue with your introduction.

The issues here have to do with the patient's decision-making capacity and the physician's desire to act in the best interests of the patient. The scenario raises some important questions. Does this patient have the capacity to make decisions about his health care? How should a physician who clearly disagrees with the patient's decision handle such a situation? Should a patient ever be forced to take a medication? I'll discuss these ethical issues in more detail.

Rule # 32   Use clear transitions between your points.

Your interviewer will do his or her best to follow what you're saying. You will undoubtedly have a number of points to make, and it's important that your interviewer stays with you. Every time you make a new point or change ideas, use transitions. The use of transition words tells your interviewer that you're moving from one point to another or when you're emphasizing something. Without transitions, your discussion can easily become choppy, or appear unorganized. Here are some examples of transitions:

- Now that I've discussed the importance of confidentiality, I'd like to move on to...
- The second point I'd like to make...
- We've look at [point # 1] but now let's move on to [point # 2]
- Finally...

I recommend that you use transitions between the introduction and first point, between each point, and before the conclusion. In the following table, you will find specific words and phrases you can use to make transitions.

Transition Words or Phrases To Help Your Interviewer Understand Your Message	
Situation	Transition words or phrases
If you need to elaborate on a point or idea	Furthermore In addition Also Moreover
If you need to transition between similar points or ideas	Likewise Similarly
If you need to transition between contrasting points or ideas	On the other hand However Conversely
If you want to show cause-effect relationship	As a result Consequently Therefore
If you want to provide an example for support	For example As an example To illustrate this
If you want to transition from the body of your discussion to the conclusion	In summary In conclusion

Rule # 33   Don't feel compelled to use all 8 minutes.

There's a belief among some applicants that points will be deducted from the interview score if the candidate does not speak for the allotted time. That's not at all true. Remember that schools are looking for evidence of the following in your responses:

- Can you apply your general knowledge to a variety of issues?
- Are you able to think on your feet?
- Can you communicate your ideas in an articulate manner?
- Can you adopt a position or viewpoint?
- Can you defend your position or ideas clearly?

So long as you demonstrate the above, you will have successfully delivered a winning response regardless of whether you speak for 5 minutes or 8 minutes. Finishing your answer before the alarm bell rings also allows the interviewer to ask you follow-up questions. In the event that your original answer was lacking in some respect, the follow-up question may allow you to bring forth important information that elevates your final interview score. If you speak for the entire time, it's possible to rob yourself of this potentially important opportunity.

Did you know...

Many interviewees have difficulty effectively addressing the issue in the allotted time. You will not be permitted to complete your answer once the bell rings. To avoid running out of time, practice making presentations in a timed manner. Note that interview rooms may not have clocks. Although you may choose to wear a watch, I've seen many applicants repeatedly check time remaining on their watch. This can affect the rapport you establish with the interviewer, and, of course, your final interview score.

Admissions Officers Speak...

"Just say what you have to say. If it takes the whole time, fine, but I will probably get bored interviewing you. Once you've said your piece, I'll ask follow up questions. The worst thing you can do is make a strong argument, then weaken it by rambling nervously trying to take up time."[4]

MMI Interviewer (Student Doctor Network)

EFFECTIVELY MANAGING TIME AT A QUESTION-BASED STATION (8-MINUTE ENCOUNTER)

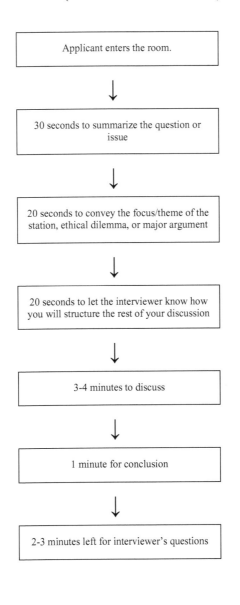

Rule # 34   Leave a lasting impression.

The most common reason for a lackluster ending is poor time management. Poor pacing often finds applicants in the middle of a sentence when the bell rings. At most MMI interviews, you will be given a warning that the interview is drawing to a close. Conclude by:

- Reviewing or reinforcing the key points or ideas you have discussed.

- Finishing with a strong sentence that links back to your introduction.

- If the question calls for it, you should have already taken a position on the issue. Restate your opinion or point of view in the conclusion.

When the interviewer has no further questions or the bell rings, you have come to the end of the interview. Let the interviewer know that you enjoyed meeting him, and thank him for his time.

Did you know...

Applicants who end their response before time runs out may be asked follow-up questions. If no follow-up questions are asked, consider what you have said so far. Is there an additional point you would like to make? Do you feel that you can elaborate on a point that you made earlier? If so, you can always say, "I was just thinking about a point I made earlier, and I realized that there's something I'd like to add. Is it okay if I bring it up now?" If you have nothing else to say, embrace the silence. Remember that there is nothing wrong with silence, and this time can be used to mentally prepare for the next station.

While going through this thought process, remember that you are being observed. Whatever you do, do not let your guard down in the remaining time that you have. There have been situations where candidates have said or done something inappropriate while making small talk. Do not feel the need to initiate small talk, but do politely engage in it if the interviewer wishes to do so. Keep whatever you say 100% positive. Remember that the evaluation form has a comments section, and anything you say or do that is viewed as concerning will be documented. Points may be deducted from your overall score, and applicants can even be removed from consideration.

> **Did you know...**
>
> Earlier we discussed the importance of making a good first impression. You also need to leave the interviewer with a good lasting impression. You can do so by telling the interviewer you were glad to meet her. Thank her for this opportunity to meet, and for considering you for one of their positions. Leave with a smile, direct eye contact, and a firm handshake if the interviewer extends her hand to you.

Rule # 35   **It's helpful to know how well you're doing in the interview. Pay close attention to the nonverbal cues of the interviewer--but recognize that there are pitfalls in this approach.**

The interviewer's body language may be your only clue as to how well you're doing. Most interviewers won't interrupt you to tell you that you're rambling. They won't tell you that your last response came across as very defensive. Better than words, their posture, movements, facial expressions, and tone of voice can indicate their reactions.

However, you should realize that MMI interviewers are instructed to give no feedback whatsoever to interviewees. Some take these instructions very seriously, and purposely stifle their nonverbal communication. They may sit rigidly in their chairs and never crack a smile. If you sense that you're losing your interviewer, try to reconnect but if your efforts don't succeed, don't get flustered. In mock interview sessions, I always tell applicants to not put too much stock in the interviewer's look and demeanor. Of course, it's human nature for us to take notice of such things but, in an MMI, you can't be sure that the interviewer's body language is a true reflection of what he or she thinks about you.

Interviewers are also asked to challenge applicants and, at times, may come across more aggressive than you would expect or like. Rest assured that they're treating all applicants in the same manner. The work of a physician is fraught with challenges and frustrations, and how you handle difficult situations in the interview setting may give the school an idea of your poise under pressure.

Medical Students Speak...

"One other thing - I thought two of my MMI interview days went HORRIBLY and I got into both of the schools. You really can't tell how you're doing, so just try to relax and have fun."

"My experiences have definitely been a lot closer to this where my raters are stone-faced and often look disinterested in what I'm saying which throws me off as I try to re-engage their interest."

"Finally, keep in mind that some interviewers may be less engaging or responsive than others. Assume that they are doing this on purpose and are trying to see how you react under stress etc. Don't let them mess with your head."[4]

Medical School Applicants (Student Doctor Network)

References

[1] AskMetaFilter. Available at: http://ask.metafilter.com/257166/Help-me-prepare-for-a-Multiple-Mini-Interview. Accessed May 5, 2015.
[2] Physicians Weekly. Available at: http://www.physiciansweekly.com/medical-training-etiquette/. Accessed May 5, 2015.
[3] Kahn M. Etiquette-based medicine. *NEJM* 2008; 358 (19): 1988-9.
[4] Student Doctor Network. Available at: http://www.studentdoctor.net/. Accessed May 4, 2015.

Chapter 10

Scenario/Acting Station Preparation

Rule # 36   **Understand what you're likely to encounter at scenario-based stations.**

At a scenario-based station, you will be presented with a difficult or challenging situation to address, navigate, or resolve. What makes this type of station even more challenging is that you will have to address the scenario by engaging in dialogue with an actor waiting for you in the room. Your interaction with the actor will be evaluated by a rater (interviewer). The following is an example of a scenario station:[1]

The parking garage at your place of work has assigned parking spots. On leaving your spot, you are observed by the garage attendant as you back into a neighboring car, knocking out its left front headlight and denting the left front fender. The garage attendant gives you the name and office number of the owner of the neighboring car, telling you that she is calling ahead to the car owner, Tim. The garage attendant tells you that Tim is expecting your visit. Enter Tim's office. Tim will be played by an actor.

Common scenarios that candidates may encounter include:

- Breaking bad news to another person
- Managing a conflict situation
- Taking responsibility for an error
- Comforting a friend, colleague, or family member in distress
- Dealing with someone who is upset

Success Tip

Reflect on your life experiences, and recall situations when you had to break bad news, take responsibility for a mistake, comfort a friend, or pacify an angry person. What did you find to be effective in those situations? What are some things that didn't work?

Rule # 37   **Empathy is important in the physician-patient relationship. Find ways to show empathy in the MMI.**

Consider the following exchange between patient and doctor:

Patient: "I have to tell you I'm in bad shape. Last few days, my knees have hurt me so much. I can hardly make it out of the house. The pain is killing me. I can't get any sleep."

Doctor: "Okay, when did it start?"

Patient: "It's been going on for some time but the last few days have been something else. If I don't get this fixed, I don't know what I'm going to do. You know how my job is. I got to be on my feet all day. If I can't work, I'm going to be in trouble."

Doctor: "I see. Does it hurt all the time?"

Patient: "It won't stop hurting. I can't even play with my grandson. It rips me apart when I tell him I can't throw the football around like we used to."

Doctor: "Have you tried taking anything for it?"

As you read the above exchange, did you feel that something was lacking in the doctor's response? The patient was sharing his concerns but the doctor seemed fixated on only gathering information. There was no acknowledgment of the patient's worries or emotions, nothing to suggest that the doctor understood the patient's concerns. Research indicates that patients are more satisfied with care when they feel a strong emotional connection with their physician. Patients are also more likely to follow through on physicians' advice and have better outcomes when their physicians demonstrate empathy.

Given the importance of empathy in the physician-patient relationship, medical schools often assess for empathy in the MMI through the use of scenario-based stations. Failure to show empathy during scenario-based stations can easily remove an applicant from further consideration. These scenarios will test your ability to remain empathetic with actors who display strong emotions. In such situations, some applicants may become frustrated and demonstrate unsuitable behavior. "At one of my stations, when the actress kept crying and I could not think of anything else to say, I tapped my lips and said to her "STOP CRYING!"[2]

Medical Students Speak...

"I had a hypothetical comfort situation in my MMI...kept changing the story to keep the conversation going into a tricky direction. Basically, every time I did/said the right thing, they moved it into a direction to try to trick me into saying something thoughtless."[2]

Breaking Bad News Scenario: Tips and Recommendations

- Use the two minutes you have before you enter the room to think about your general approach.

- As you process the information, ask yourself whether the person is or isn't expecting bad news.

- If the person is expecting bad news, begin your conversation by finding out how much he or she already knows. This will allow you to assess how much the person understands, and his or her emotional state.

- Prepare the person for the bad news with an appropriate phrase.

  - "I have some sad news to share with you."
  - "There's no easy way to say this but..."
  - "I just received a call from..."

- Come right to the point. This is not the time for small talk or speaking in a roundabout manner.

- Always look the person right in the eye.

- Be gentle in your approach.

- Avoid rigidity in your approach. Show flexibility and adaptability as you respond to the actor's cues.

- Give an account of what has happened so that the person understands.

- Expect to encounter emotions. These may include anger, shock, disbelief, sadness, or distress. As emotions arise, react appropriately to them. Acknowledge and address these emotions. "I can see that you're really upset about this."

- If they respond with intense emotions, such as anger, remain calm. If they cry, be there to comfort them.

- If the recipient remains silent, don't feel compelled to fill up the silence. While letting the news sink in, simply sit with them in a sympathetic manner.

- Decide the next action step when the time is right.

Managing Conflict Scenario: Tips and Recommendations

- Use the two minutes you have before you enter the room to think about your general approach. In any conflict situation, remember that your goal is not to win but rather find a solution that is satisfying to both parties.

If it's your fault...

- If it's an obvious issue where you have erred, then you have to acknowledge your error and apologize.

- In your apology, let the other person know that you understand the problems that have resulted from your words or actions.

- Do not make excuses or offer explanations. Simply take full responsibility for your error and inform the other party of your intent to resolve the situation.

- If you are not sure how to rectify the situation, consider several options, present them, and come to some agreement on which is best.

If it's not clear where the fault lays or if both parties share blame...

- Start by informing the person of why you wish to speak, the issue at hand, and how you feel. Phrase feelings with "I" rather than "You." "I feel ___ when you..." is better than "You make me ___..."

- Listen carefully to the other person's perspective. Avoid interrupting. After hearing the person's point of view, restate it in your own words to make sure you understand both views.

- Conflict often arises from miscommunication, incorrect assumptions or incomplete information. For example, we may assign motives for someone's behavior based on incorrect assumptions.

- By listening carefully, you are better able to understand where the other person is coming from. Don't be afraid to ask questions to better understand the other person's perspective.

- As you discuss the situation, don't overreact. If the other person is angry, allow him to vent his anger.

- Even if you feel angry, remain poised and calm. Choose your words carefully, avoiding any language that may further inflame the situation.

- Propose some solutions, and invite the other party to do the same. Discuss these in more detail, and come to some compromise. If you're unable to find a solution, consider meeting again to continue the discussion.

- Remember that your goals are to resolve this conflict by finding a fair solution. If it's someone you must continue to work with, do what you can to preserve the relationship.

Dealing With An Upset Person: Tips and Recommendations

- Set the stage for the encounter. "Is it okay if I sit next to you? We can talk about what's happened, and the best way for me to help you."

- Begin by acknowledging how the person appears to you. "You seem to be very upset."

- Ask the person to tell you what happened, how they feel, and how you can best help.

- Allow the person to speak without interrupting.

- Make appropriate eye contact.

- Show that you are actively listening. "Uh-huh" and "Go on" invites the person to continue.

- Reflecting out loud what has been said shows that you have understood the person. "If I understand you correctly, you're really concerned that…"

- Use a calm voice.

- Don't offer false reassurances. Applicants sometimes have the tendency to say, "It is okay. Everything will be alright." The problem with this statement is that you don't know that for sure. Therefore, it's best to refrain from making such reassurances.

- "I know how you're feeling. I've been in the same situation." These words may seem empathetic to you but can be very irritating to the person. When people are acutely distressed, hearing that others have gone through similar situations doesn't feel comforting.

- Some applicants resort to humor to diffuse the emotional tension. There may be a role for humor later but right now the emphasis should be on acknowledging and respecting how the person is feeling and helping him handle it.

- Recognize that your approach should not be rigid. Show flexibility and adaptability as you respond to the actor's cues.

- Expect to encounter other emotions. These may include anger, shock, disbelief, sadness, or distress. As emotions arise, react appropriately to them. Don't get to a point where you can no longer accept the emotion.

- If they respond with intense emotions, such as anger, remain calm. If they cry, be there to comfort them. You may be tempted to give the person a hug but not everyone responds positively to touch in these situations. You may feel that touch shows genuine concern and willingness to help but some people will find it awkward or even uncomfortable.

- Decide the next action step but don't hurry it. Decision-making can be difficult for a distressed person.

Rule # 38   Avoid clichés.

In role playing scenarios with mock interviewees, I've come across a number of clichés and statements that may seem appropriate but could easily be taken the wrong way. I would urge you to avoid these statements.

Statements To Avoid In Scenario-Based Stations (Comfort/Bad News)	
Statement	**Reasons To Avoid**
You have to be strong now.	It's not helpful to tell someone who is grieving that they shouldn't grieve anymore. People have to express their grief before the healing process can begin.
I know exactly how you feel.	Even if you've suffered a loss, you can't know exactly how the person is feeling. Relating what they are going through to something you've experienced takes the focus off of them and places it onto you.
You need to put this behind you.	The grieving process can take varying amounts of time.
Everything happens for a reason.	After a loss, it's difficult for people to believe that what occurred is part of a grand plan.
He/she is in a better place now.	Many people believe that those who suffered before passing away are now in a better place. However, not everyone shares these beliefs.

Dos and Don'ts For Scenario-Based Stations	
Do...	**Don't...**
Acknowledge how the actor is feeling	Reveal your own discomfort with the situation
Validate the actor's experience	Tell the actor how you think he should feel or urge him to get over it
Be patient and allow the actor to speak	Fill up the silence, even if you're feeling uncomfortable or the actor's taking too long to respond.
Ask the actor questions	Admonish the actor for not getting over the emotion
Encourage the actor to take whatever time is necessary to deal with his feelings	Talk about how you felt when you were in a similar situation. The focus should be on what the actor is going through and how he feels.

Rule # 39   **Ask for specific feedback following scenario-based station practice**

The following evaluation form can be used to provide valuable feedback about your scenario-based station performance during mock interviews.

Feedback Evaluation Form for Scenario-Based Station		
Statement	Yes	No
I greeted the actor warmly.		
I sat, leaned in, and adopted an open, receptive posture.		
I gave the actor my undivided attention.		
I listened to the actor without interruption.		
I encouraged the actor to share his feelings.		
I acknowledged the actor's feelings in an empathetic way.		
I validated or confirmed the legitimacy of the actor's feelings.		
I communicated empathy for the actor's feelings through my words.		
I showed empathy through my nonverbal behavior (e.g., nodding, looking concerned, etc.)		
I invited the actor to share his ideas and viewpoints (thoughts, worries, feelings, expectations) before making any suggestions.		
I was approachable, friendly, and respectful.		
I showed genuine concern for the actor.		
I sought to determine the next step or action based on partnership.		

Medical Students Speak...

"The first was an actor that played the part of a mentally disabled teen that needed me to teach him how to tie his shoelaces. It was pretty challenging especially because the actor's role was to get very frustrated and verbally upset during the process. I couldn't have prepared for this scenario at all other than remembering to stay calm, act with kindness, and do my best to keep 'teaching' him how to tie his shoes."[3]

References

[1]Eva K, Rosenfeld J, Reiter H, Norman G. An admissions OSCE: the multiple mini-interview. *Med Educ* 2004; 38 (3): 314-26.
[2]Student Doctor Network. Available at: http://www.studentdoctor.net/. Accessed May 4, 2015.
[3]Mindful of Medicine. Available at: http://mindfulofmedicine.com/2014/12/28/med-school-interviews-mmi/. Accessed June 3, 2105.

Chapter 11

Task/Collaboration Station Preparation

Rule # 40   **Task-based stations test your ability to stay poised under pressure while working as part of a team to complete a complex task.**

At a task-based station, you will be asked to complete a task, often with another applicant. The Stanford University School of Medicine offers the following description of a task station:[1]

Two applicants participate in a scenario in which one applicant is asked to perform a complex test (such as assembling or repairing a model) with the other applicant giving directions for dealing with or assembling the model.

When you enter the room, there will be two raters, one of whom will be responsible for observing and rating your performance. The second rater will be tasked with evaluating the other applicant. Task stations are used to learn more about an applicant's teamwork, problem solving, and communication skills.

The task will often be complex, difficult to complete within the time allotted, or even impossible. Emily Aaronson, a graduate of the McMaster University Michael G. DeGroote School of Medicine, recalls a particularly memorable task-based scenario she encountered. After entering the room, she found two chairs placed back to back. She was asked to sit in one while another person sat in the other. Both were given a piece of paper covered in small dots. "My partner's dots were numbered and mine were not," said Ms. Aaronson. "He had to talk me through how to connect the dots." Later, she discovered that the dots on each page were not identical. "My knee-jerk reaction was, 'Are you kidding me?'"[2] Faced with such a daunting task, applicants under pressure to complete the task in a time-limited manner may demonstrate behaviors and attitudes considered unsuitable in future physicians.

Rule # 41   **Prepare for the task-based station by delivering instructions to someone else.**

Now that you know the type of situation you may encounter in a task-based scenario, practice by performing similar tasks with a partner under the same conditions. Some examples include:

- Print out the instructions to build a paper airplane. Then arrange the furniture so that you and your partner are sitting back to back. Give your partner a blank piece of paper, and guide him through the process of making the paper airplane.

- A similar exercise can be done with origami. Origami instructions and designs are easily available on the Internet, and it's not necessary to have origami paper. Start with easy to make shapes and then challenge yourself with harder designs.

- Use Lego models. Give instructions to your partner on how to build a Lego model. You can sit back to back, and your partner should not see the model. He will take direction from you.

If you're giving instructions...

- Inform your partner of the task ahead of you. "The point of this exercise is to build a paper airplane..." Check to make sure your partner understands the task.

- Set the stage for a positive encounter by encouraging your partner to ask for clarification or help whenever needed. "If anything I say is unclear, please tell me."

- Indicate that you will break down the task into a series of small steps.

- Before taking an action step, make sure your partner is holding the paper, model, or other prop the same way you are. In other words, identify the present position and orientation of the prop before providing the first set of instructions. Then do the same after each step is completed.

- If you sense that your partner is frustrated, offer words of encouragement and support. Show empathy. Remember to be nonthreatening if you must repeat instructions or correct a misstep. Be tactful and delicate when you point out a mistake.

- Encourage your partner to provide updates on his progress and when the step has been completed.

Rule # 42   **Prepare for the task-based station by receiving and following through on instructions given by someone else.**

If you're receiving instructions in a task-based scenario, much of your success will hinge on your ability to listen carefully. Over a century ago, Sir William Osler uttered a dictum which is arguably his best-known saying. "Listen to your patient, he is telling you the diagnosis." Although these words continue to have as much meaning today as they did then, research indicates that physicians are lacking in their listening skills. "Studies show that the clinician's ability to explain, listen and empathize can have a profound effect on biological and functional health outcomes as well as patient satisfaction and experience of care," writes the Institute for Healthcare Communication. "Further, communication among healthcare team members influences the quality of working relationships, job satisfaction and has a profound impact on patient safety."[3]

If you're receiving instructions...

- Your partner will be giving you instructions periodically. Remember to let your partner speak without interruption.

- Offer facilitating remarks to indicate that you are listening. Examples include "Uh-huh" and "Go on."

- There may be times when your partner is silent. Perhaps she is thinking about the best way to explain something. Silence often feels uncomfortable, and it's common for people to fill it up with words. However, a good listener is comfortable with silence.

- After receiving instructions, provide a recap to your partner to ensure that you have correctly understood the instructions.

- If you sense that your partner is frustrated, show empathy. Offer words of encouragement and support.

- Remember to be nonthreatening if you must ask for the instructions to be repeated or clarified. If you have questions, ask your partner one question at a time.

- Provide your partner with updates on your progress and when the step has been completed.

Rule # 43   **Ask for specific feedback following task-based station practice**

The following evaluation form can be used to provide valuable feedback about your task-based scenario performance during mock interviews.

Feedback Evaluation Form for Task-Based Station (Giving Instructions)		
Statement	Yes	No
I gave an overview of the task that we were expected to accomplish as a team.		
I encouraged my partner to ask for clarification or help if needed.		
I listened with an open mind to my partner's point of view.		
I acknowledged and appreciated my partner's efforts, and provided encouragement during the task.		
If my partner was frustrated or had an issue with me, I listened and carefully considered his point of view without becoming defensive.		
I kept an open mind to my partner's ideas even if he disagreed with me.		
I offered empathy during the encounter when needed.		
I acted as a positive role model for collaboration and teamwork.		

Feedback Evaluation Form for Task-Based Station (Receiving Instructions)		
Statement	Yes	No
I listened to my partner without interruption.		
I restated the instructions to make sure that I correctly understood my partner.		
I asked for clarification if needed in a gentle manner.		
If I had questions, I asked one question at a time.		
I acknowledged and appreciated my partner's efforts, and provided encouragement during the task.		
If my partner was frustrated or had an issue with me, I listened and carefully considered his point of view without becoming defensive.		
I offered empathy during the encounter when needed.		
I acted as a positive role model for collaboration and teamwork.		

Did you know...

As the founder of F Cancer, Yael Cohen deals with the emotions of cancer on a daily basis. She learns so much about her employees during times of hardship. "Everyone we hire works for free as an intern for a month first and I will give them tasks that are impossible on purpose just to see what happens. Do they lose their s---? Do they blame themselves? Do they take it out on someone else? You need to see what happens when they fail. As a team, we're going to fail. As individuals we're going to fail."[4] That's precisely what task-based MMI stations are designed to assess – your ability to remain poised at times of great stress.

References

[1]Stanford School of Medicine. Available at: http://deansnewsletter.stanford.edu/archive/11_08_10.html. Accessed May 4, 2015.
[2]The Globe and Mail. Available at: http://www.theglobeandmail.com/life/interview-20-theres-no-easy-way-to-ace-this-one/article1344084/. Accessed May 4, 2015.
[3]Institute for Healthcare Communication. Available at: http://healthcarecomm.org/about-us/impact-of-communication-in-healthcare/. Accessed May 3, 2015.
[4]99U. Available at: http://99u.com/articles/7247/want-better-employees-give-them-an-impossible-task. Accessed May 22, 2015.

Chapter 12

Preparing for Other Types of MMI Questions

For many students, the MMI equates to scenarios and discussion questions. However, medical schools often devote one or more stations to traditional interview questions and behavioral interview questions.

For example, the prompt on the door may just ask a single traditional interview question. "Why do you want to be a physician? Enter the room and discuss your response with the interviewer." With these types of stations, your response should of course be shorter, allowing time for follow-up questions and a back-and-forth conversation.

Although you may be expecting traditional interview questions, we've found that many applicants still provide standard, generic responses. And this is a big mistake.

A standard, generic response represents a lost opportunity. Why? If instead you can provide a unique, memorable response--one that highlights your outstanding qualities as well as your fit with this particular medical school--you will stand out and be remembered.

We've found that many students just don't take the extra time and preparation needed to create these unique responses. Instead, many rely on discussion forums and blog posts and craft their responses based on what they find there. For interviewers, it can sometimes seem like an entire day of generic response after generic response. As one interviewer reported, "It is an essential station, however after 40 candidates I found it a little tedious."

How can you elevate your responses?

First, it's important to reflect on all your previous activities and experiences. These can provide significant insight into your strengths, interests, and goals.

Next, it's important to do a deep dive into this particular medical school. What is the mission of the school? What is it known for? What are unique opportunities offered by this medical school that are not offered elsewhere?

Traditional Interview Question Example: What are your strengths?

I've asked this question in many interviews, and I often hear back that the student is "a hard worker, a team player, and would come to work every day willing to work with others and get things done."

Contrast that response with this one:

I'm a hard worker and I'm very persistent. When I was elected the community service lead of our pre-medical society, I spoke to the leadership of our local healthcare system. I'm very interested in rural healthcare, and they were excited to hear about my proposed project to bring student volunteers to their rural clinics on a weekly basis. Although they agreed to the project, it took a year of back-and-forth communication, and much paperwork, to launch the project. I'm really glad I persisted, though, because now our students have the opportunity to volunteer at the clinics, and the nurses and patients with whom we've worked have told me how much they appreciate the student volunteers. I know I'm going to need that same hard work and persistence in medical school, and I'm ready and excited.

This particular response was crafted for the Texas A&M University Medical School, whose website lists the school's three primary missions on the very first page. One of these missions is to improve disparities in rural healthcare. For a student who has experience and an interest in this area, this medical school is a great fit--and she needs to highlight that in her responses whenever possible.

For more guidance on traditional medical school interview questions, please see an example of how a student provides a generic "before" answer and then crafts a much stronger "after" response in Chapter 19.

Our companion book, *The Medical School Interview: Winning Strategies from Admissions Faculty,* is devoted to helping you craft responses to traditional interview questions.

We also offer our signature course, Medical School Interviewing 101, where we teach applicants how to quickly and confidently prepare for their traditional medical school interview with our expert strategies. The course includes a series of before-and-after videos and our expert step-by-step approach.

Our goal is to help applicants go from good to great to unforgettable. For more please see TheInterviewCourse.com.

Behavioral Interview Questions

What are behavioral interview questions? Examples include:

- Tell me about a time when you faced criticism
- Tell me about a time when you had a conflict with a coworker
- Tell me about a time when you faced and overcame a challenge

These have also been referred to as "past behavioral questions." Situational questions ask applicants what they would do in a hypothetical situation, while behavioral interview questions ask what their actual experience was. Studies in non-medical admissions have demonstrated similar reliability and acceptability for both types of questions.[1]

Proponents of this type of question believe that past behavior helps predict future behavior. They've been used in the business world for years, and now they're becoming more common in the medical school interview.

In order to best prepare for this type of question, it's really important to spend significant time reflecting on your past experiences. That's because it can be very challenging to come up with a great example on the spot.

In answering these questions, it's important to highlight a real experience. It's also important to choose a real experience in which you acted in a mature, professional manner.

Another important point: the question is not actually "tell me about a time when you had a conflict." The question should actually read "tell me about a time when you had a conflict and tell me what you did to handle it."

As you reflect on your prior experiences, it can be very challenging to find the right examples. It's very much like Goldilocks. You don't want one that's too hot or too cold. In other words, you don't want an extreme example (it got so heated that we both got expelled) and you don't want a blip of an example (my roommate and I couldn't agree on where to go for dinner).

The right example would be one where there was an actual conflict that caused you concern or distress, and in which you were able to deal with a conflict in a mature, professional manner.

Apart from finding the right example, it's also important to structure your response in the correct way. One helpful strategy is to use what's known as the STAR response.

- Situation: Describe what happened
- Task: Describe the task
- Action: What steps did you take to deal with the situation?
- Response: What was the outcome?

We've provided several sample responses to behavioral interview questions in Chapter 18. Below we've provided examples of other behavioral interview questions.

Examples of Behavioral Interview Questions

1. Tell me about a time when you displayed teamwork.
2. Tell me about a time when you showed initiative.
3. In your college years, how did you handle conflict? I'd like to hear about a specific example.
4. Tell me about a time when you worked effectively under a great deal of pressure.
5. Tell me about a particularly stressful situation you encountered in college and how you handled it.
6. Tell me about a time when you were forced to make an unpopular decision.
7. Tell me about a time when you were disappointed in your performance.
8. Tell me about a situation in which you overcame adversity.
9. Tell me about a time when you had a difficult communication problem.
10. Tell me about a problem you had with a classmate or professor. How did you handle it?
11. Tell me about a time when you handled a stressful situation poorly.
12. Tell me about a time when you became really angry over a situation in college.
13. Describe to me a situation in which you had to break someone's confidence.
14. Tell me about a time when you witnessed unprofessional or unethical behavior on the part of a classmate. How did you handle it?
15. Tell me about a time when you had to build rapport quickly with someone under difficult conditions.
16. Tell me about a difficult decision you've made in the last year.
17. Tell me about the major challenges you've faced in your college career.
18. Give me an example of a time when you motivated others.
19. Give me an example of when you showed initiative and took the lead.
20. Tell me about a time when you were able to successfully work with another person, even when you didn't like them personally.
21. Tell me about a time when others working with you disagreed with your ideas. How did you handle it?
22. Tell me about a time when you had to go above and beyond the call of duty in order to get a job done.
23. Describe a situation that required a number of things to be done at the same time. How did you handle it? What was the result?
24. Tell me about a time when you put your needs aside to help a classmate or coworker understand a task. How did you help him or her? What was the result?
25. Describe a situation in which your performance did not meet your professor's or supervisor's expectations. What happened? How did you handle the situation?
26. Tell me about a time when you said something or did something and then later realized it was wrong.
27. Tell me about a time when you worked in a group and it did not go smoothly.

Examples of Behavioral Interview Questions

28. Tell me about a time when you were responsible and helped others.
29. Tell me about a time when you interacted with people who held different views than you did.
30. Describe a situation where you made a mistake and what happened afterwards.
31. Name a time when you helped improve a process.
32. Tell me about a time when you did everything you could and the outcome was still a failure.
33. Tell us about a time when you tried your hardest but you failed.
34. Name a time when you worked with a team and overcame an obstacle.
35. Tell me about a time when someone came to you with a problem that you empathized with.
36. Describe an encounter you had with someone that was unpleasant and how you handled it.
37. Name a time when you caught a small problem and fixed it before the problem became larger.
38. Tell me about a time when you stood up for a person in need.
39. Tell me about a difficult situation you encountered in your clinical experience and how you handled it.
40. Tell me about an ethical decision you faced and how you handled it.

References

[1]Yamada T, Sato J, Yoshimura H, et al. Reliability and acceptability of six station multiple mini-interviews: past-behavioural versus situational questions in postgraduate medical admission. *BMC Med Educ*. 2017;17:57. doi:10.1186/s12909-017-0898-z

Chapter 13:

Task Completion

Case #1

For this exercise, you will be working with a partner. You will be handed a single instruction sheet, while your partner will be given a single blank piece of paper. In the room, you will be seated on chairs, back-to-back. Your task is to instruct your partner to complete the project. You will have five minutes to complete the project.

Sample Answer

Student 1: Hi partner, I'm Mary. The instructions I've been given are for a paper plane. Are you ready to start?

Student 2: Hi Mary, I'm Sarita, and I'm ready to go.

Student 1: Great. The instructions are not written out. It's basically an illustration with a whole bunch of arrows, so it might take me a little bit at some of the steps. I just wanted to give you a heads up on that. I'll be going through the directions step-by-step. Also, if you have any questions as we're working through this, please let me know.

Student 2: Absolutely, will do.

Student 1: OK, for step one, I need to clarify. Is your piece of paper a standard 8 1/2 x 11 printer paper sheet? And is it white on both sides?

Student 2: Yes, and yes.

Student 1: And are you right-handed?

Student 2: Yes, I am.

Student 1: In that case, I'm going to have you hold the paper in your right hand with the long end running horizontally.

Student 2: Done. I'm now holding the paper in my right hand, running horizontally.

Student 1: OK, for this next step I'm going to have you take the top left corner and fold it downwards towards you until it reaches the bottom edge of the paper. Then, I'm going to have you firmly crease it.

Analysis

She introduces herself and describes the task. "We will be making a paper airplane."

She made it clear that these were not going to be written instructions, and that there were times when she might be silent while figuring out the directions. She also asks her partner to ask any questions if needed.

She made sure that she and her partner were oriented in the same way. "Please hold it with the long end running horizontally."

Student 2: Just to confirm, I should now have a large, folded triangle taking up the left side of the paper?

Student 1: Yes, that's correct.

Student 2: OK, that's done now.

Student 1: Great, now for step two you will...

The applicant receiving instructions did a good job of updating her partner on her progress. "Done."

Chapter 14:

Challenging Scenarios, Acting

Case #1

You are the nurse manager on a busy hospital floor. One of your nurses is upset after a difficult patient encounter. The patient was in considerable pain but the nurse was unable to give him anything because the next dose of pain medication was not scheduled for another several hours. As she tried to explain the situation, the patient became quite angry and questioned the nurse's dedication to her profession. Hurt by this, the nurse lost control of her emotions, and the situation escalated with the patient requesting to speak with the nurse manager. The patient is now waiting for you in the room.

Sample Answer

Nurse Manager: Hello Ms. Smith. I'm the nurse manager on the floor. I understand you wanted to speak with me. How are you feeling?

Patient: Terrible. I'm in a lot of pain and no one seems to care.

Nurse Manager: Can you tell me what happened?

Patient: I just want some medication to help me with this pain. It's now so bad – nine out of ten. I've just been sitting here hoping and waiting for medication. The nurse told me that if I calmed down, that I may feel better. Can you believe that? I need some pills or even a shot. I need something. I'm really hurting.

Nurse Manager: So, let me see if I've understood the situation. You're in a lot of pain, and you don't feel like the current pain medication is providing you with enough relief.

Patient: Yes, that's what I'm saying. I need something stronger than what I'm getting. I told the nurse this, and she kept telling me to calm down. I asked her to help me, and she kept telling me that it wasn't time for the next dose. I asked her to call the doctor, and she didn't look too happy about that.

Nurse Manager: It sounds like you would find it helpful if I reached out to your doctor. That's something I can do. I will call and let him know that your pain medication is not keeping the pain under control. Perhaps he can make an adjustment to your medication or stop by and take a look at you.

Analysis

In a MMI scenario with an angry person or patient, sit if you can. Sitting gives the person the feeling that this is important to you and that you have the time to address it.

The nurse manager invites the patient to tell her how he's feeling and describe the events that transpired. Listening patiently to an angry patient or person will often help defuse the situation. Remember to let the person talk.

No matter how difficult the person is, you must be professional in your interactions. Although you may not agree with his comments, refrain from responding with your own harsh comments.

To ensure that she has understood the situation, the nurse manager provides a summary and looks for corroboration. It is clear that she now understands the source of the patient's concern.

Sometimes patients will offer a potential solution. If it's reasonable or appropriate, you can agree to it. If no solutions are offered, ask the patient what he would like for you to do.

Perhaps he can make an adjustment to the medication or stop by and take a look at you.

Patient: I would love that. I don't know why it's so hard to find the doctor.

Nurse Manager: Let me go and call the doctor. Let's see if we can come up with a plan to address this. How does that sound to you?

Patient: That sounds wonderful.

Nurse Manager: Before I take care of that, I wanted to see what else I can do for you. I know you're uncomfortable, and I apologize for that. Is there anything else I can do to help you? Are you cold? Do you need a blanket? How about a snack?

Understanding that the situation has been difficult for the patient, the nurse manager looks for ways to make the patient feel comfortable.

Patient: Would you mind turning the TV on for me?

Case #1: Key Points

In any unhappy or angry person scenario, you can utilize the mnemonic BLAST to diffuse the emotions and resolve the situation.

Using the BLAST Mnemonic with Angry or Unhappy Patients	
B	**Believe** in the patient's concern and distress, even if the patient is irrational, incorrect, exaggerating, or lying.
L	Actively **listen** to the patient. Allow the patient to vent. Remain calm and be sure your nonverbal communication communicates attentiveness and understanding. Show understanding by clarifying and repeating the patient's concerns.
A	**Apologize** to the patient. This does not mean you to have accept responsibility if you didn't do anything wrong. You are simply apologizing to the patient for what he's going through.
S	**Satisfy** the patient by offering several solutions.
T	**Thank** the patient for sharing concerns, and the opportunity to make things better.

From Dermatology Times. Mnemonics help to keep patient satisfaction levels high. Available at: http://dermatologytimes.modernmedicine.com/dermatology-times/content/tags/aesthetic-procedures/mnemonics-help-keep-patient-satisfaction-levels-?page=full. Accessed May 12, 2015.

Case #2

You are the doctor in a busy medical practice. Today, you are running 1.5 hours late. Earlier in the day, a patient came to see you, and you realized that she was having a heart attack. Concerned for her, you stabilized the situation, made arrangements for transfer to the hospital, and called the cardiologist to let him know of the patient's situation. Your next patient is waiting for you. Before you enter the room, your nurse informs you that he is very angry about waiting so long to see you.

Sample Answer

Patient: You're finally here.

Doctor: It sounds like you're feeling frustrated.

It's very important to acknowledge a patient's emotion.

Patient: I've been waiting for well over an hour. When I spoke to your office staff this morning, I told them that I needed my blood pressure medication refilled. They told me that you wouldn't be able to refill it unless I came in to the office. I told her about my busy day, that I would be leaving for an overseas trip tomorrow. That didn't seem to matter to her. Then when I got here, I asked the receptionist if they knew whether you were running behind schedule. She looked at me and said she had no clue. How rude is that?

No matter how difficult the person is, you can't take what he's saying personally. Remember to listen and communicate with respect. Above all, guard against saying anything negative even if the situation escalates.

Doctor: Well, it sounds like my front office staff didn't give you the information you were looking for.

Although you will feel the pressures of time, you will score points for listening. By letting the actor say what he must say, you're showing the interviewer that you're a patient listener.

Patient: No. They didn't. Was I really asking too much? All I wanted was some idea of how long you would be so I can plan my day better. I'm leaving for this last-minute work trip. It's going to be stressful, and on top of that I'll be missing my daughter's birthday. I was hoping to spend some time with her before I left.

Don't forget the importance of body language. If you're saying the "right things" but your nonverbal communication says something entirely different, points may be deducted from your interview score. Nonverbal behaviors to avoid include crossing your arms, scratching your hands or face, tapping hands against your lap, or shaking your foot.

Doctor: I know you've waited a lot longer than you wanted to. Then you tried hard to find out when I would see you but the staff didn't tend to your concerns. I can see how upsetting that would be, especially with you getting ready for a trip, and having to miss your daughter's birthday. I know how much your daughter means to you.

Analysis

Patient: I just thought that I could be in and out of here quickly. I mean, it's just a refill. Now my day is all out of whack.

Doctor: You know how hard I try to stay on schedule. What I can never predict is when I may encounter a patient emergency. It just so happened that earlier today, I saw a patient with a severe medical emergency. I had to do a lot to get her stabilized and in a safe place. That's what made me so late for your appointment. I do apologize for making you wait as long as you have. Your time is precious, and important to me. I hope you can understand why things happened the way they did today.

Patient: Boy, I had no idea. I sure hope that your other patient does okay. Thanks for explaining everything to me.

Long wait times are a common cause of patient anger. How should anger be addressed in such situations? In one study, participants were shown a video tape of an angry patient and asked to rate 12 physician responses. Highest scores were given to an apology combined with an explanation of the reasons for the delay.

References

McCord R, Floyd M, Lang F, Young V. Responding effectively to patient anger directed at the physician. *Fam Med* 2002; 34 (5): 331-6.

Case #3

As the manager of on an electronics superstore, you are in charge of 10 employees. One of your employees, Larry, has been receiving and sending texts regularly during work hours. He has even done so while providing service to customers. Today, you noticed that a customer became visibly upset when Larry pulled out his cellphone in the middle of their conversation. You are puzzled by Larry's behavior because up until this started two weeks ago, he had been one of your best employees. You have decided to discuss the situation with Larry. Larry is waiting for you in your office.

Sample Answer

Manager: Thanks, Larry, for meeting with me today. Lately, I've noticed that you've been using your cellphone during the workday. You've been sending and receiving texts, even in front of customers. Today, one of our customers was upset when you checked your phone. Is there a reason for this behavior?

Larry: I'm very sorry. My wife and I are really concerned about my son. You see, he's been skipping class, and getting into fights. We had to sit him down to talk, and things really didn't go well. My wife's taking this especially hard, and I wanted to reassure her that everything will be fine. I'm also concerned about my son. I don't want anything bad to happen to either one of them.

Manager: Thank you for sharing all that with me, Larry. It does sound like you're going through a lot at home. This must be a very difficult time for you, and I certainly hope that everything works out. If you'd like to take some time off to resolve these issues, that would be just fine with me. Just let me know.

Larry: I appreciate your support. I think that would be a good idea. Some time off may be just what I need to get things back on track.

Manager: Meanwhile at work, I believe it's important for all of us to deliver the highest quality customer service. Can I ask you to please leave your cellphone in your locker during the workday? Of course, I don't mind at all if you take it out during lunch or breaks.

Larry: That sounds fine to me.

Analysis

Notice how the manager focuses on Larry's actions at work rather than Larry as a person. This approach makes it less threatening for Larry, and increases the chances that this will be a productive exchange between the two parties.

Here the manager expresses concern for Larry, recognizes that this is a trying time in Larry's life, and expresses hope for a positive outcome.

After providing support, the manager returns to the work issue at hand. Here she offers a possible solution.

Manager: Larry, you've always received high marks for your customer service. We appreciate the ways in which you make our customers feel special, and that's what we're looking for in our team members. You know that you're a big part of the impression that we make on our customers, and it's crucial that we provide the service that our customers want. Do you feel that this is a reasonable request?

Larry: Yes. It's quite fair. I had no idea that my texting was causing so many problems. I guess I was so caught up in what's been going on at home. I promise you, from now on, I'll keep my phone in the locker. I'll only access it during breaks.

The manager now reaffirms her faith in Larry. At the end, she seeks Larry's input and confirmation.

Although the manager was able to arrive at a definitive solution in this case, remember that some MMI situations may not have a solution. If you're involved in such a scenario, you will be mainly evaluated on your ability to show empathy and make the actor feel comfortable enough to discuss the situation with you.

Case #4

You are an employee working in the shoe section of a major department store. A customer returns to the store upset about a problem with shoes she bought five weeks ago. The store policy allows for returns with full refund within 30 days of purchase. For older items purchased from the store, employees can issue store credit, exchange items, or arrange for repair when items are defective.

Sample Answer

Employee: Hello. My name is _____. How can I help you today?

Customer: I bought these shoes for my daughter's prom. Yesterday, when she tried them on, the heel immediately broke. It's three days before prom and my daughter is so upset because she doesn't have shoes.

Employee: You must be very upset. I'm so sorry this happened.

Customer: Well, sorry won't cut it. My daughter's prom is a big deal, and she's upset about the shoes. How does a heel break when it has never been worn? What kind of shoe department is this? You should be concerned about quality.

Employee: I'm going to do whatever I can to make this right for you.

Customer: I'm just so angry. I really didn't need this.

Employee: You know, I would be too if I were in your position. Is it okay if I ask you a couple of questions? Let me start by asking you when you bought these shoes? Do you have a receipt?

Customer: Yes, I have a receipt. I bought these shoes, let me see, it looks like five weeks ago.

Employee: I see. According to this receipt, it has been about five weeks since your purchase.

Customer: That's what I said.

Analysis

In any MMI scenario where you have to interact with an actor, focus entirely on the actor. Do not concern yourself with the rater who will be sitting in the corner of the room evaluating your performance. Remember that your goal is to connect with the actor.

Acknowledge emotion and express belief in what the person is feeling or saying. This helps to build trust.

Allow the person to vent their feelings.

These can be intense encounters but you must remember to remain calm and composed. Maintain eye contact, remain attentive, and offer expressions of understanding.

Employee: I can imagine how upsetting this is for you. I'm sure you have so much to do for your daughter's prom, and you didn't need this to happen.

Customer: Yes. There's a lot to do, and I want to make this prom a special day for her.

Employee: So, you bought these shoes five weeks ago. Your daughter tried them on yesterday, and the heel broke. You only have three days before prom and you need shoes before then. You must also be concerned about whether these shoes are returnable.

Clarify and repeat back what you've heard to show the person you truly understand the situation.

Customer: Yes, I am.

Employee: Well, I wish we could refund your money. But our store's policy only allow for full refunds within 30 days of purchase. Here's what I can do for you though. I can give you credit for the shoes that you can apply to another purchase or allow you exchange them for another pair. Another option available to us is repair of the heel. Of course, this would be at no expense to you. Which would you prefer?

You should explore possible solutions but don't agree to something that you can't offer. At some point, you may need to call on someone else to help you resolve the situation. Remember that a physician should be able to recognize his limitations, and call upon others if need be.

Customer: If I had the heel repaired, would it be available before the prom date?

Employee: Yes. We have a relationship with the shoe repair service in this mall. If you give me the go ahead, I'll take these shoes myself to their store, and make sure they're ready for you in two days.

Customer: That would be great. Let's do that.

Case #5

Your patient returns for check of his blood pressure. For the past year, you have been making adjustments to the patient's blood pressure medication. Although the patient has not developed any problems related to the high blood pressure, you have been worried about the toll the blood pressure is taking on the patient's body. You are specifically concerned that he may develop a heart attack, stroke, or kidney disease. You have prescribed medication to control the blood pressure and reduce the risk of problems related to it. Unfortunately, efforts to control the blood pressure have not been successful. Today, the patient's blood pressure remains high. Before entering the patient's room, the nurse informs you that he hasn't been taking his blood pressure medication. Enter the room and talk to the patient about why he hasn't been taking his blood pressure medication.

Sample Answer

Doctor: I see that your blood pressure is still high today. The nurse was telling me that you haven't been able to take your medication. Are you having a problem taking it?

Patient: It's not good to be off the medication. I should be taking it.

Doctor: Is there something that concerns you about the medication?

Patient: I've never been keen about taking medication. I keep hoping that if I exercise and eat right that I won't need to take the medication.

Doctor: So it sounds like you don't like the idea of having to take medication. Are you worried about side effects?

Patient: It's something to think about but it's more the thought of taking medication.

Doctor: Before we discuss this, I thought we could take some time to review some important points about high blood pressure. I'd like to start by asking you a question. We've talked about the importance of controlling blood pressure in the past. Do you know why it's so important?

Patient: You told me about the dangers of blood pressure. I know it can damage my heart or even cause stroke.

Doctor: That's right. High blood pressure can lead to heart attacks, kidney disease, and stroke. Do you know why I've recommended medication to control your blood pressure?

Analysis

Note that the interviewee has broached the topic in a nonjudgmental manner. The encounter is more likely to be productive if the patient does not feel threatened. Open-ended questions are best at first.

Patients who are noncompliant with treatment often feel guilty, self-conscious, defensive, or ashamed. Blaming or accusing the patient may inflame the situation.

To effect change in behavior, it's important to first understand if the patient recognizes the importance of the medical problem, and the health risks if the problem is untreated.

Patient: The medication can control my blood pressure, and that would cut down my risk of running into problems.

Doctor: You're absolutely right. What we have tried so far hasn't been working. I'm concerned about what high blood pressure can do to your health. What do you think?

Use of "we" shows the patient that this is more of a partnership rather than the doctor imposing his viewpoint on the patient.

Patient: I know have to get more serious about this. I don't want to develop any problems.

Doctor: Let's get back to what you said earlier. You were hoping that diet and exercise would help lower your blood pressure.

Patient: That's why I don't always take the medication. I keep hoping that diet and exercise will do the job.

Doctor: What can I do differently to help you with this?

Asking the patient for his thoughts to address the problem builds a stronger partnership.

Patient: I've tried diet and exercise for so long. I think it's time for me to give the medication a real chance.

Case #5: Key Points

- In a meta-analysis of compliance in common conditions, such as diabetes and high blood pressure, researchers found that only 59% of patients take medication as prescribed most of the time.
- Noncompliance is a major cause of treatment failure, and is not often appreciated by physicians.
- If the MMI asks you to engage in a dialogue with an actor playing the role of a noncompliant patient, remember to be gentle and nonthreatening in your approach. Many noncompliant patients feel guilt, embarrassment, or a sense of failure. These are strong negative emotions, and your ability to show concern for the patient will be the key to a successful encounter.
- Avoid blaming or accusing the patient with such statements as "You're not doing a good job taking your medication." Contrast this with "I'm concerned that if we don't get your blood pressure under control, you could develop some problems with your heart." Statements starting with the word "I" and expressing your concern set the tone for partnership to solve the problem.

Approach to the Noncompliant Patient

Step 1: With any noncompliant patient, be gentle in your approach. To understand its root cause and solve the problem, discuss noncompliance in a nonjudgmental manner. Use open-ended questions to begin the dialogue.

Step 2: Assess the patient's understanding of the medical problem, and risks to health if the problem is not treated.

Step 3: Determine if the patient has any concerns or questions about the recommended treatment.

Step 4: Determine if the patient has been considering or using other treatments.

Step 5: Make noncompliance a shared problem.

Step 6: Ask the patient about strategies that he believes might be effective.

References

Cramer J, Benedict A, Muszbek N, Keskinaslan A, Khan Z. The significance of compliance and persistence in the treatment of diabetes, hypertension and dyslipidaemia: a review. *Int J Clin Pract* 2008; 62 (1): 76–87.

Kleinsinger F. Working with the noncompliant patient. *Perm J* 2010; 14 (1): 54–60.

Case #6

You are a pediatrician, and a mom brings in her son for his 4-month check-up. He received all his vaccinations at birth and at his two-month exam. At the end of the appointment, when you tell the mother her child is scheduled to receive several vaccinations, she expresses hesitancy. She does not want her child to receive these because of concerns on sudden infant death syndrome and autism. You are aware that there is no scientific evidence linking vaccines to either condition. Enter the room and counsel the mother on vaccinations for her child.

Sample Answer:

Doctor: We want to make sure your baby stays healthy, which is why we've scheduled these vaccinations. Before I tell you more, I want to make sure I understand your concerns and questions so that we can discuss them further. Can you tell me more about your concerns?

Mother: I've read about the link between vaccines and sudden infant death syndrome. I don't want my son to die.

Doctor: I can understand that it would be very scary to read that. Can you tell me more about where you read that?

Mother: It was in an article on a medical website, but I don't remember exactly which one. It just scared me so much.

Doctor: I can only imagine how scary it would be to read that. And when you're trying to be a good parent, it can be very challenging to be faced with all of these conflicting claims on the internet. Would it be OK with you if I shared some information with you based on my own experience?

Mother: Yes, I'd really like to hear what you've heard.

Doctor: To start with, I'm so grateful that we have vaccines available. It's easy to forget how serious and even deadly some of these diseases can be, because most people today have never seen children with polio or whooping cough, but these cause very severe illnesses in children. In fact, I still remember treating an unvaccinated child with measles. He had to be hospitalized, and it was very

Analysis:

It's important to elicit more information about the mother's concerns.

The doctor empathizes with the mother's concerns. She is respectful and honors the patient's goal of trying to be a good parent. She asks permission before sharing her own experience and recommendations.

She shares her own experience to put the focus on the dangers of the disease.

scary. Luckily, he pulled through, but it just made me so grateful to know that vaccines would keep other children safe from the dangers of these diseases.

In this office, we've vaccinated thousands of children, and I have never experienced a severe, serious side effect with any of my patients. I can also assure you that these vaccines have been extensively tested for safety. Many, many studies have been conducted and have shown no link between sudden infant death syndrome and vaccines.

The doctor has empathized with the mother, but provides her own experience on vaccine safety and emphasizes the safety testing that's been done.

Mother: I sort of get what you're saying. And my son was just fine after his previous shots. But what about vaccines and autism?

Doctor: There's been a lot of research in this area also, and there is just no scientific evidence to suggest a link between vaccines and autism. In fact, I plan to vaccinate all of my children. These vaccines will help us get your baby ready for a long, healthy life.

The doctor includes her own personal decision to reinforce her recommendation.

Mother: I'm just not sure. Can I think about it for a while?

Doctor: How about we go ahead and schedule a vaccination appointment for next week? That way, you'll have some time to think, and when you come in next week we'll be ready to proceed if you're ready. If you have any questions in the meantime, you can let me know.

The doctor makes the vaccine appointment the default option.

Case #6: Key Points

Note in this answer how much active listening the physician engages in before providing her own (strong) recommendations. As we've all now learned with COVID vaccines, it can be incredibly challenging to counter medical misinformation.

There is clearly no one approach that works with all parents. One technique that has been studied is called motivational interviewing. In this technique, the physician starts by building a trusting, respectful relationship. This involves asking open-ended questions and listening as the parent shares their concerns. Most parents are trying to make decisions based on their concerns for their child's safety and well-being, and the physician here has verbalized that she understands that this is the mother's goal. After that, the physician asks for permission to share information. The goal is to avoid belittling or condescending to the patient.

Once the parent has given you permission to share information, it's helpful to share personal experiences as well as the research. The parent here is concerned about sudden infant death syndrome and autism, two conditions frequently described on social media as linked to vaccines. It is important to assure patients that scientific evidence does not support this association, and that vaccines are safe.

Using your personal experience, such as vaccinating your own children or explaining that you have not experienced adverse events in your own patients, can help support and strengthen your recommendation.

It's also helpful to focus on the dangers of disease, not just on the potential side effects of vaccines.

Patients may still be ambivalent or resistant to vaccines. It is important to leave the opportunity for future conversations on vaccinations open. This may take the form of scheduling another appointment upfront or providing the patient with additional information such as pamphlets or online resources.

Chapter 20 provides an example of vaccine hesitancy related to COVID vaccination.

References

[1].Price S. Talk to Patients About: Vaccines and SIDS. *Tex Med.* 2021;117(2):43.

[2.]Centers for Disease Control and Prevention. Talking with Parents about Vaccines for Infants | CDC. Published April 1, 2019. Accessed July 19, 2021.   https://www.cdc.gov/vaccines/hcp/conversations/talking-with-parents.html

[3.]Centers for Disease Control and Prevention. Prepare for Vaccine Questions Parents May Ask | CDC. Published November 18, 2019. Accessed   July   19,   2021. https://www.cdc.gov/vaccines/hcp/conversations/preparing-for-parent-vaccine-questions.html

[4.]Price S. Talk to Patients About: What's Wrong With Vaccine Exemptions? *Tex Med.* 2020;116(5):47.

Chapter 15:

Challenging Scenarios:

Discuss How You Would Handle the Case

Case #1

Physician burnout is recognized as a serious threat to physician well-being, as well as the quality of medical care provided in the United States. In fact, recent legislation has allocated a significant amount towards burnout prevention strategies.

You have been appointed to a national committee to study this issue and make recommendations. What are some measures that you would like to either study further or institute?

Sample Answer:

As a premed student, I've read about the risks of physician burnout. I've also had long discussions on this topic with my mentor, Dr. Katta, who shared with me how this topic has affected her friends and colleagues. I was very heartened to see that our government is taking this issue seriously by funding burnout prevention measures.

As a member of a national committee, I would focus my efforts on three main areas. The first area would be on digital tools, the second would be on physician support programs, and the third would be on structural issues contributing to burnout.

In terms of digital tools, I have read that current electronic medical record systems may be contributing to burnout. I would allocate some of our funding to studies of current use of these systems, especially focusing on feedback from physicians. Some of our funding would then be used to improve the systems, with a focus not only on patient care, but also on the users of the EMR.

In terms of programs that support physician well-being, I would focus on studying these first. In speaking with my mentor, she commented that some of her colleagues have found that some burnout prevention programs have not been very helpful. So I would allocate a portion of our funding to studies of evidence-based interventions that have been shown to improve physician well-being in the inpatient setting and the outpatient setting. If certain programs were shown to help, I would focus on funding these.

Analysis:

This student provides a strong introduction, discussing how he has read about this topic and has had discussions with his mentor.

This is a strong positioning statement, outlining three areas that he would focus on.

He makes a strong point here that he would first focus on studying the impact of burnout prevention programs, and only then would he implement those that were shown to be evidence-based interventions.

The third area I would study would be structural factors that might be contributing to physician burnout. For example, I know physicians have to complete certain checklists for Medicare patients. I would study the trade-offs of these kinds of requirements. Are these truly improving patient care or healthcare savings, and if there is a trade-off in terms of physician burden, is that trade-off worth it?

This is a significant issue and there are obviously no easy answers, but I would start with researching these three areas as a first step.

This concluding sentence reiterates his position that he would start by researching these three areas.

Case #1: Key Points

Burnout has been defined as "emotional and exhausting conditions related to the working environment."

The Three Domains of Burnout:

- Emotional exhaustion
- Depersonalization
- Low personal achievement

Research indicates that the United States is experiencing an epidemic of physician burnout. The prevalence has been estimated as close to 50% among practicing physicians, as well as those in training. This is extremely concerning, as it has been long recognized that physician burnout is associated with impaired patient care, including a higher risk of medical errors. The risks to physicians themselves are significant.

Work-related stressors are a major risk factor for physician burnout. These stressors include

- Excessive workload
- Excessive work hours
- Excessive burden from record-keeping
- The use of electronic medical records
- Inefficient work processes
- A hostile work environment
- Organizational factors
- Others

In one review article, interventions to reduce burnout were focused on two main categories.

- Physician-directed interventions that focused on individual measures
- Organizational-directed interventions that focused on the work environment

A number of interventions have been studied and have been shown to be successful in reducing factors that contribute to physician burnout.

Interventions that Reduce Factors in Physician Burnout:

- An 8-week mindfulness course followed by a 10-month maintenance course

- A family medicine program in which medical assistants performed initial work-ups (which included history-taking and education on preventive care). This permitted physicians to focus on physical examination and medical decision-making. This intervention improved burnout rates from 53% to 13%.

- Professional coaching to increase efficacy and strengthen professional skills

- A mental health training program consisting of a brief course

---

Burnout can be measured through validated surveys, and institutions are starting to recognize the importance of addressing physician burnout and instituting measures to prevent and mitigate it.

Ultimately, burnout prevention is an incredibly important issue in healthcare. Our workforce needs to be supported in every way possible in order to ensure a healthy workforce and in order to provide the highest quality of patient care.

References

Patel RS, Sekhri S, Bhimanadham NN, Imran S, Hossain S. A Review on Strategies to Manage Physician Burnout. Cureus. 2019 Jun 3;11(6):e4805. doi: 10.7759/cureus.4805. PMID: 31404361; PMCID: PMC6682395.

West CP, Dyrbye LN, Erwin PJ, Shanafelt TD. Interventions to prevent and reduce physician burnout: a systematic review and meta-analysis. Lancet. 2016 Nov 5;388(10057):2272-2281. doi: 10.1016/S0140-6736(16)31279-X. Epub 2016 Sep 28. PMID: 27692469.

Case #2

You are an internal medicine resident physician working with a medical student. You enter the room of a newly admitted patient with the medical student, who is African American, to watch the student perform a physical examination. A few minutes into the encounter, the patient requests to see someone other than the medical student. As the resident physician, how could you approach this situation?

Sample Answer:

I would begin by asking the patient why they would like to see someone other than the medical student. Given the medical student is African American in this scenario, it would be easy to assume the patient does not want to be examined by the student because of their race. However, this is not necessarily the case, and to handle the situation correctly, I would need to make sure I have a good understanding of what is going on. For example, the patient may not want a medical student examining them, and patients have the right to refuse to be seen by a medical student.

If the patient did answer they did not want to be examined by the medical student due to a racial or other bias, I would tell the patient about my confidence in the medical student's skills and firmly, but gently, explain to the patient what constitutes unacceptable behavior in this encounter. If the patient continued to press, it may be a good idea to remove the medical student from the situation and call in a more experienced clinician.

Following the encounter, I would speak to the medical student in private, and help provide or connect them with resources. If the patient did not want to see the medical student because the student is African American, I would check on how the student was doing and affirm what they experienced was discrimination.

Analysis:

The student is careful not to jump to conclusions. It is always important to ask questions and reach a clear understanding of the situation.

The student is providing a strong, clear answer to the prompt. "Remove the medical student from the situation and call in a more experienced clinician."

This is an important part of the response. After the acute patient care situation was handled, it is important to discuss the situation with the student and offer support and resources.

Finally, I would consult with an experienced attending physician, either bringing them into the room if the encounter became exceedingly uncomfortable, or at the very least reporting what happened and consulting with them on next steps. It may even be worthwhile to consult with a hospital ethics committee.

The use of transition words such as "finally" strengthens the response.

In summary, I would first make sure I properly understand the situation by speaking with the patient and asking what is wrong, careful not to make assumptions. Then, I would try to deescalate the situation in the room, and if needed, call in a more experienced attending. Finally, I would check in with the medical student afterwards.

This is a strong concluding statement.

Case #2: Key Points

Notice that in this response, the student first tries to get more details from the patient. To properly handle this situation, the resident physician would need to fully understand it. This helps avoid assumptions. It is important to recognize patients have a right to refuse care from a medical student and asking the patient more questions in this case helps clarify whether this is the patient's concern.

One way of dealing with racial bias against healthcare workers is by expressing your own confidence in your colleague's or student's talents, while also making it clear to the patient that discrimination is unacceptable. At the same time, it is important to keep the situation under control and respectful, and seek the help of another colleague, for example an attending, if needed.

It is essential to check in with the colleague or student who experienced a racist encounter and offer to debrief. By telling the colleague or student that you felt the encounter involved overt racism, they are less likely to doubt this behavior was unacceptable and feel supported.

References

1.   Garran AM, Rasmussen BM. How Should Organizations Respond to Racism Against Health Care Workers? *AMA Journal of Ethics*. 2019;21(6):499-504. doi:10.1001/amajethics.2019.499

2.   Annas GJ. *The Rights of Patients: The Basic ACLU Guide to Patient Rights*. Springer Science & Business Media; 1992.

Case #3

Near the end of a 24-hour shift, you realize that your fellow intern is in a state of distress. During rounds, the supervising physician asked her to begin a blood pressure medication on Mr. Smith. Several hours after writing the medication order, she realized that she wrote the order in the wrong patient chart. By the time she caught her mistake, the nursing staff had already administered the medication to Mr. Jones. After receiving the blood pressure medication, his blood pressure fell and IV fluids had to be given to normalize the blood pressure. After she tells you what happened, she urges you to not share this information with the supervising physician. Discuss how you would handle this situation.

Sample Answer

From what I gather, this is a case involving an intern who has made a medical error. Her intent was to treat a patient with a blood pressure medication. Unfortunately, the wrong patient was given the medication, and he suffered a drop in his blood pressure. Fortunately, the blood pressure improved with fluids. After making this mistake, the intern is understandably upset. She is urging me not to share this information with our superior. Do you feel that I have a good understanding of the situation?

Seeing how distressed she is, I would begin by offering her emotional support. I'd let her express her feelings for as long as she needs to, and acknowledge how she's feeling. When it's appropriate, I would tell her that we all make errors. I might even share with her some of my own errors so that she realizes that she isn't alone. I would hope that through this conversation she would realize that it can be difficult to admit fault but it shows that we are responsible and caring physicians.

After offering her my support, I would ask her why she doesn't want to discuss this withs the supervising physician. She may be concerned about her grade. Perhaps she really needs a recommendation from our supervising physician. There may also be concerns about what impact this mistake may have on her future job prospects. She may be fearful that our attending physician would be harsh and judgmental rather than supportive. I would remind her that our attending physician is ethically and legally responsible for our patient's care. If we don't tell him what happened, he can't do

Analysis

By providing a summary of the case, the interviewee demonstrates an understanding of the situation. He invites the interviewer to correct any misunderstandings on his part. This is an effective way to make sure you're headed in the right direction.

The discussion continues with an emphasis on the intern's emotional well-being. It's clear that the interviewee is showing empathy. Empathy is defined as the ability to imagine what it's like to be in another person's situation.

He tries to place himself in the intern's shoes, and comes up with a number of reasons for the intern's reluctance to share the error. The interviewee recognizes that the intern has an ethical duty to inform the supervising physician of the error. He knows that the patient should come first.

his job properly and that has the potential to impact the patient's care.

Plus, there's a good chance he's going to learn about it. If he does, it will be a lot worse than if we bring it up. It's one thing to make an error. It's a very different thing to hide it. If we do hide it, it'll raise questions about our reliability, trustworthiness and character.

I would also say that disclosing the error to our attending physician allows for a discussion about the reasons why the error took place. From this, we can learn how to perform better as individuals and also identify ways to avoid such errors in the future.

Failing to disclose the error has consequences that extend beyond patient care.

In conclusion, I believe that it is important for my fellow intern to inform our supervising physician of this error in patient care.

The interviewee raises a very important point about learning from errors.

Case #3: Key Points

- When a physician colleague makes a patient care error, there should be concern for both the patient and physician.
- Although physicians have a professional duty to address errors with colleagues, research indicates that this often does not occur.
- Begin such conversations in a gentle and non-confrontational manner. "I was hoping to talk with you about Mr. Smith's care. There's something that I'm concerned about. Do you have time to talk about it?"
- Remember to be emotionally supportive. This is undoubtedly an emotional time, and your support can help set the tone for the ensuing conversation.
- Try to delicately uncover professional or personal (high stress, depression, relationship issues, family issues, substance abuse) factors that may have led to the error.
- Explore ways to prevent such errors in the future, and discuss the importance of disclosure to superiors and patients.

How Do Residents Respond to Mistakes Made in Patient Care?

In a survey of over 250 internal medicine residents, researchers asked participants about major mistakes made in medical care, and how they responded to these errors:

- The mistake was discussed with the supervising attending physician in only 54% of cases.
- Residents discussed the mistake with the patient or patient's family in only 24% of cases.
- 5% of residents reported not telling anyone about the error.
- Making an error in patient care was emotionally distressing for residents.
- 81% of residents reported feeling remorseful.
- 72% of residents reported feeling guilty.
- 60% of residents reported feelings of inadequacy.
- 79% of residents reported feeling angry.

Wu A, Folkman S, McPhee S, Lo B. Do house officers learn from their mistakes? *Qual Saf Health Care* 2003; 12: 221-8.

Case #4

At a party, you're surprised to see one of your physician partners. He is on call but is at the party with a glass of wine in hand. As the evening progresses, your colleague continues to drink and it's clear that he is now tipsy. Having taken call before for your group, you know how busy it can be, and you worry about your colleague's ability to provide care to patients in this state. How would you handle this situation?

Sample Answer

My biggest concern would be the danger my impaired colleague presents to our group's patients. I would also be concerned about what's going in my colleague's life and his overall mental state. Drinking on call is obviously not the best choice, and raises concerns about his emotional well-being. This is a very difficult situation with the potential to impact the lives of our patients, my colleague, and, of course, myself.

Before I took any action, I would need to be sure that patients are at risk. Although it appears that he is under the effects of alcohol, I would need to confirm this. There's a lot at stake here – the health of our patients, and his reputation, livelihood, and privacy, my relationship with him, and what others might think.

I'd also worry about the repercussions of my actions as it relates to my own career. If I pursue this, there is a possibility that I may damage my relationship with him. The partners in the group may be forced to take sides, and some may be very disapproving of the choices that I make. I could be accused of having my own agenda, and this could all affect my career.

Although my actions could threaten my own career, nothing would trump the dangers to patient care that this situation presents. I would have a duty to prevent harm and protect patients from impaired colleagues. There may also be legal precedents requiring me to report my impaired colleague.

I could also see that intervening now in my colleague's health might allow him to fix

Analysis

The interviewee shows concern for the safety of her group's patients. She also expresses concern for her colleague. She recognizes that her actions or inactions could have a significant impact on all parties involved.

Since so much is at stake, she takes a cautious approach.

She considers the potential harm to her own career.

Although the situation poses risk for her professional career, she indicates that she will place patients above everything else.

things before it got even worse. He may not see it that way of course.

In terms of how I would handle the situation, I would take immediate action. I would urge the colleague to have me or one of my partners take call for him. If he doesn't agree, I would notify our chief medical officer or partners to arrange for someone else to cover him. I would ask our office to review any calls that he received from patients to make sure that no harm will come to them from his actions.

She now addresses the key question, "How would you handle this situation?" Again her position shows that patients come first.

After preventing immediate harm, I would talk with my colleague. I would encourage him to seek help. If he agrees and follows through, then I would support him. If not, I would have to contact the chief of service and seek guidance on how to proceed. Perhaps there is a program in the hospital to help physicians struggling with these issues.

She continues to show concern for her partner's emotional well-being and expresses the desire to help him. She's even willing to take it a step further if he does not agree to seek assistance. Research indicates that a significant percentage of doctors feel unprepared to report or deal with an impaired colleague.

The bottom line is that I would do whatever is necessary to ensure that our patients received the best possible care.

Case #4: Key Points

- Impairment may occur because of a physical, mental, or substance-related disorder. The end result is interference with the physician's ability to deliver safe patient care.
- A physician who is concerned about an impaired colleague has an ethical and legal responsibility to address the issues. Failure to do so puts the safety of patients at risk.
- Once impairment is recognized, meet with the physician to offer support and share concerns. This conversation should not become a personal attack or confrontation. Remember that impairment affects everyone, including the physician, his or her family, colleagues, and, of course, patients.
- Discuss potential options with the impaired physician.
- If the physician is not open to any reasonable option, it may be necessary to notify the clinic, practice, or hospital where the physician practices. States and licensing boards may have reporting requirements, and physicians should be familiar with these guidelines.

References

Mossman D, Farrell H. Physician impairment: When should you report? *Current Psychiatry* 2011; 10 (9): 67-71.

Yancey J, McKinnon H. Reaching out to an impaired physician. *Fam Pract Manag* 2010; 17(1): 27-31.

DesRoches C, Rao S, Fromson J, Birnbaum R, Iezzoni L, Vogeli C, Campbell E. Physicians' perceptions, preparedness for reporting, and experiences related to impaired and incompetent colleagues. *JAMA* 2010; 304 (2): 187-93.

Case #5

Mr. T, a 75-year-old Mandarin-speaking man, has just been diagnosed with colon cancer. The son asks the doctor to not disclose the diagnosis to his father. He maintains that people from China of that generation are not told they have cancer. The son says Mr. T will lose hope if he's told he has cancer. How would you handle this situation if you were the physician?

Sample Answer

To begin with, I would like to summarize the case to make sure I fully understand it. This is a difficult situation in which a patient has been diagnosed with cancer. The physician has been asked to not inform the patient of this new diagnosis. The family indicates that people of their father's generation from China are not told of a cancer diagnosis. There is concern that the patient may lose hope if he's told that he has cancer. Do you feel that I have a good understanding of the situation?

This case really brings up some important issues, including trust in the doctor – patient relationship and how cultural values can impact the way in which physicians care for patients. I would like to discuss these issues, and then end with how I would approach this particular situation.

The first point I'd like to make is that trust is essential in the doctor – patient relationship. Lying and deception undermine trust, and I would worry that not being truthful to the patient would make him feel that he has been betrayed.

However, I recognize that there are cultural issues in play here. In some cultures, it might be standard practice to not disclose a diagnosis of cancer or other serious illness. Disclosing the information may cause the patient to suffer, and I can see how some patients would be more hopeful if information was withheld. Even in a culture, there will be some people who would want to know, and I think that's the key here. Would this patient want to know?

Analysis

Begin with a summary of the case. Check in with your interviewer to make sure you have a good grasp of the situation. This will increase the likelihood that you will address salient points.

In the introduction, provide the listener with a blueprint to follow. The interviewer now knows the issues that will be discussed, and the order in which the information will be presented.

Be on the lookout for cultural issues in the MMI. The United States has a multicultural population, and our physicians must be sensitive to different cultural beliefs and practice.

Never assume that all patients would behave in the same manner.

There are other situations in which I might not share information. If a patient was severely depressed or suicidal, I might worry about the consequences of disclosure. In these cases, I would consult with psychiatry to assess likelihood of harm. If the patient was a danger to himself, I might wait until his mental health improves.

If I were the physician, I would ask the patient how he would like me to proceed. Would he like to know the diagnosis or would he prefer that I discuss the diagnosis only with his family? If the patient said, "I don't want to know," I would have to respect his wishes.

In summary, I think that there are many reasons to tell patients the truth. I believe most patients in the U.S. would want to know so that they can understand treatment options, ask appropriate questions, and make informed decisions about their health. However, I do recognize the importance of being sensitive to patients' cultural beliefs and practices, and I would take that into account in my decision-making.

It's important not to be too rigid during the MMI. In medicine, there are often exceptions that need to be made based on the situation.

Many interviewees end their response with a whimper rather than a bang. Close with a strong summary statement.

Case #5: Key Points

- In some cultures, families withhold bad medical news out of concern that disclosure will lead to feelings of despair in patients.

- Since the United States is such a culturally diverse nation, physicians will sometimes encounter situations in which families make requests outside of the norm.

- Truth telling, as highlighted in this case, is one such example. In this case, the patient's son felt that it was his responsibility to protect the patient from distressing news.

- This poses problems for physicians in the United States who are accustomed to having patients make their own health decisions. Physicians prefer to keep patients informed so that they can make educated decisions about their health (patient autonomy).

- Such situations require physicians to be sensitive and delicate in their approach. It's important to show respect for the perspectives of all family members.

- Ask family members about their concerns. What do they fear will happen if the patient is told the truth? Although the family may want to protect their loved one, the patient may wish to be actively involved in the process. It's never wise to assume that everyone within a culture would want to be treated the same way.

- Determine what the patient would like. It's up to the patient to decide whether he wants to be involved in the decision-making.

Case #6

A 38-year-old banker informs his physician that he recently tested positive for HIV. "Doc, you have to promise me not to tell anyone. I don't want to lose my job." The physician urges the patient to disclose the diagnosis to his wife. After a long conversation, the patient adamantly refuses to do so. "Doc, this will end my marriage," he says. How should the physician proceed?

Sample Answer

In this situation, the patient recently discovered he was positive for HIV. He is concerned that this information may be shared with others. He is worried about losing his job. He also fears that telling his wife will destroy his marriage. This brings up important issues related to patient confidentiality. Among the points I'd like to address are the importance of confidentiality, consequences of breaking a patient's trust, and reasons why physicians may have no choice but to do so.

I'd like to begin by discussing why confidentiality is so important. At the heart of the physician-patient relationship is trust. Trust may be lost when personal health information is divulged without the patient's consent. If there is lack of trust, patients may be less inclined to seek care and share important health information. This could certainly affect the quality of care delivered.

Although personal health information should only be released if the patient provides consent, I believe that there are several exceptions to this rule.

The first exception involves concern for the safety of others. I believe that a physician may have to breach confidentiality if the patient informs the physician that he or she intends to harm others. In these situations, the physician's duty to prevent harm trumps the mandate to maintain confidentiality.

Confidentiality must also be breached when there is a legal requirement to do so. I know that, with some communicable diseases, physicians are required to notify the public

Analysis

The interviewee provides a summary of the case, and identifies the key issue (confidentiality). The last sentence in this paragraph gives the listener an idea of where the interviewee will take the discussion.

Note the interviewee's use of transition statements ("I'd like to begin..."). These help the interviewer process the information more easily.

Interviewee recognizes that there are limits to confidentiality.

With every ethical scenario involving patient confidentiality, always be vigilant for exceptions to the rule which would require physicians to breach confidentiality. The exceptions fall under concern for the safety of others and legal requirements.

health department. In these cases, the physician has a duty to protect public health, and this duty supersedes the mandate to maintain confidentiality.

In this case, I believe that the physician has compelling reasons to not maintain confidentiality. First, I would worry about his wife being infected with HIV. If she knew that her husband was HIV-positive, she could take proper steps to protect herself from harm. Second, if a diagnosis of HIV requires notification of public health authorities, I would be legally mandated to inform them.

Interviewee now returns to the question posed in the scenario.

I realize that my actions would have serious consequences for my patient's life. For that reason, I would explain all of this to the patient in a sensitive and respectful manner. It would be my hope that we could come to some agreement. I would do my best to address his concerns, and support him. In terms of his job situation, I don't see why I would need to disclose this to his employer in the banking industry.

If you must break confidentiality, be straightforward with the patient. Let the patient know that you're obligated to do this, and offer reasons why this is the case. Offer an apology, and then the opportunity for the patient to disclose the information on his own. If the patient refuses, then inform the patient that you must disclose the information.

In conclusion, I believe that physicians should maintain confidentiality. However, there are some exceptions to this rule, and this case is a good example of that.

Challenge Questions for Confidentiality

Is it ever appropriate for the physician to breach confidentiality?

With every ethical scenario involving patient confidentiality, always be vigilant for exceptions to the rule which would require physicians to breach confidentiality. The exceptions fall under concern for the safety of others and legal requirements. If there are no exceptions, then always maintain confidentiality.

What if a family member wants to discuss the patient's health?

If you're presented an ethical scenario where a family member is asking about their loved one's health, remember to seek permission from the patient before disclosing any personal health information. If, however, the patient has suffered an injury or illness and can't make his or her own medical decisions, then the physician may discuss the situation with the next of kin. The physician will need a family member to make informed decisions on the patient's behalf. Appropriate individuals would be those named in a living will or healthcare power of attorney.

What if the patient is an adolescent?

Trust in the physician-patient relationships is important to adolescents. Many adolescents are afraid that their health concerns will be disclosed to their parents. These fears can prevent adolescents from seeking care, sharing sensitive information, and returning for follow-up. In one study of adolescent girls, nearly 60% reported that they would cease to use sexual health services or delay testing/treatment for sexually transmitted illnesses if this sensitive information was divulged to parents (Reddy). Laws regarding confidentiality with adolescents vary from state to state. In some states, sensitive issues (sexually transmitted illnesses, contraception, pregnancy) can be kept confidential if the patient is able to provide informed consent.

What if you have to break confidentiality?

If you must break confidentiality, be straightforward with the patient. Let the patient know that you're obligated to do this, and offer reasons why this is the case. Offer an apology, and then the opportunity to disclose the information on their own.

For more information on patient privacy, please see Chapter 17 on Basics of Medical Ethics

References

Reddy D, Fleming R, Swain C. Effect of mandatory parental notification on adolescent girls' use of sexual health services. *JAMA* 2002; 288 (6): 710-14.

Case #7

Mr. N is a 35-year-old patient who is concerned about his weight. As the years have passed, he has put on considerable weight, and now weighs nearly 250 pounds. He has tried a variety of diets and exercise regimens without success. He recently read about a Chinese herbal supplement that has shown amazing results. You are not familiar with the supplement but are concerned about potential side effects. You have had other patients who have developed side effects after taking supplements. In some cases, there have been some worrisome interactions between herbs and prescribed medications. Discuss the issues involved, and how you would handle the situation.

Sample Answer

Losing weight is difficult for so many people. With this patient, it seems that he has tried different diets and exercise programs. I'm sure he's concerned about obesity and its associated health risks. I'm sure that he's also frustrated by his inability to lose weight. I can see why he would explore other options. It seems that he is hopeful that an herbal supplement may help him reach his goal.

First, I would tell the patient that I'm glad he's taking such an active interest in his health, and researching possible treatments. I know that some patients may be reluctant to share their thoughts of taking an herbal supplement with their doctor so I would be very gentle in the way that I discussed this with him. I would ask him how he came to learn about the supplement, and if he knows others who have used it.

I would then take the time to review all of his prior efforts to lose weight. I would patiently listen to his story, and inquire about the factor or factors that he believes prevented him from reaching his goals. If there were some options that we hadn't explored in terms of conventional medical therapy for weight loss, this would seem to me a good time to discuss them.

If he felt strongly about the herbal medication, I would be honest with him and tell him about my lack of experience with the supplement. I would ask him to give me some time to research it. I would remind him that herbs may also have side effects, and we would need to make sure there are no interactions with other medications he takes.

Analysis

Complementary and alternative medicine (CAM) is defined as practices that are outside of mainstream or conventional medicine.

Recent studies have shown that CAM use is common, especially by patients having chronic conditions. Forms of CAM include, but are not limited to, naturopathic medicine, homeopathy, Ayurveda, and traditional Chinese medicine. Perhaps the most common form of CAM is the use of herbal products.

Doctors are encouraged to make decisions based on available research. However, CAM research is very much in its infancy, and there is much we don't know about its efficacy.

It's clear that our patients are turning to CAM, and therefore it's important to engage in dialogue with our patients about this important issue. Doctors should avoid dismissing or ridiculing CAM therapies because it can certainly affect the patient relationship.

Any consideration of therapy must take into account the risk of harm and potential benefits. A CAM therapy that does not appear to be harmful can be harmful if it prevents the patient from utilizing established and effective treatment.

Once I reviewed what we know about the supplement, I would present this information to him and let him know if I think it would be safe to take. If he chose to take it, I would monitor him very carefully for side effects.

Case #8

You are working in the emergency room, when a patient is brought in following a serious car accident. The paramedic informs you that the patient is a Jehovah's Witness. She has sustained serious injuries, with severe bleeding, and may require a blood transfusion. What do you do?

Sample Answer

I know that physicians are sometimes faced with these types of challenging scenarios. When I was volunteering in the emergency room, I noticed that the ER nurses would ask every patient about their wishes regarding potential blood transfusions.

In this case, the most important thing would be the emergent care of the patient. Can I stop the bleeding and stabilize the patient without having to use a blood transfusion? If a blood transfusion is deemed medically necessary, can I administer that blood transfusion in a patient whose faith speaks against the use of blood transfusions?

To begin with, I would try to determine the patient's own wishes. Patient autonomy is such an important ethical principle, and I would do everything in my power to try to understand the patient's wishes. Hopefully, they are conscious and coherent and are able to tell me in their own words.

If they were not able to convey their wishes, I would then do everything possible to see if there was any other indication of their wishes. I especially would not want to jump to any conclusions about a patient's wishes. I know that among practitioners of different religious faiths, there are variations in how closely individuals adhere to the tenets of their faith, and therefore I would try to understand everything I could about the patient's own wishes.

I would look through the chart to see if there was any information there. I would check to see if there were any advanced directives about blood transfusions. If this information wasn't available, I would check with their

Analysis

The student includes their own personal experience with this issue.

This is a strong opening, focusing on "the most important thing."

The student introduces the important ethical principle of patient autonomy.

It is important not to jump to conclusions regarding a patient's wishes, and the student makes it clear that she understands that religious practices, even within a particular faith, may vary.

She is describing her search for collateral sources of information.

family members or loved ones to try to understand their wishes.

If I could not locate any information in a timely fashion, I know the most important thing in an emergent situation is to treat the patient, and therefore I would proceed with blood transfusion if it were medically necessary. If I had enough time, I would definitely try to speak with the hospital administration and legal team. If we didn't have enough time, I would make sure to document thoroughly, because there may be legal ramifications. After the patient was medically stabilized, I would then make sure to speak with the hospital administration more thoroughly.

She has described a systematic progression of what she would do. She has also considered the need for documentation.

This is a tricky scenario, and it really highlights the importance for patients of trying to prepare advanced directives to make sure that their wishes are known in a medical emergency. It also highlights how important it is for physicians providing routine care to help their patients understand the need for advance directives, and especially how important these become in a medical emergency.

She ends with a strong conclusion and highlights the need for advance directives.

Important Information about Jehovah's Witnesses

There are over 1 million Jehovah's Witnesses in the United States. The Jehovah's Witness society is a Christian denomination. It traces its origins back to 1872.

In charge of the society is a governing body known as the Watchtower Society. Witnesses believe in a very strict and literal interpretation of the Bible. It is this interpretation which leads practitioners of the faith to refuse some types of medical care.

For example, one passage from Genesis reads "but you must not eat blood that has its lifeblood still in it." This passage has been taken to mean that blood cannot be eaten as a form of nourishment.

In medicine, we can "nourish" our patients in different ways. One form of nutrition is delivered through the IV or intravenous route. Since blood transfusions are also given intravenously, the Watchtower Society views blood transfusion as a form of nourishment, or eating of blood.

This view led to a 1945 church decision, and that decision prohibited Jehovah's Witnesses from receiving blood transfusions. Many Jehovah's Witnesses believe that by accepting blood, they will give up their right to be a member of their faith and lose any hope of eternal life. In the past, the Watchtower Society has supported the shunning and social isolation of members who violate this doctrine.

In 2000, the Watchtower Society loosened its stance a bit, backing off on the excommunication of members who violate the doctrine. They wrote, and I quote, "If a baptized member of the faith willfully and without regret, accepts blood transfusions, he indicates by his own actions, that he no longer wishes to be one of Jehovah's Witnesses. The individual revokes his own membership by his own actions."

It's important to have this context and background about Jehovah's Witnesses, because we hear so much about how we shouldn't give blood transfusions to practitioners of the faith.

Case #8: Key Points

A strong response to this scenario requires an understanding that practitioners of religious faiths may vary in how they observe their faith, as well as an understanding of the major ethical principles underlying the practice of medicine.

Not all practitioners of this faith refuse blood transfusion in all cases. Especially in an emergent situation, it's important to ensure that the patient understands the consequences of refusing blood transfusion. It's not unheard of for a patient to go against this tenet of their faith when faced with a medical threat to their life.

There are four major ethical principles that underlie the practice of medicine:

- Autonomy
- Beneficence
- Non-maleficence
- Justice

In general, autonomy takes precedence over beneficence. In other words, a patient can decline medical care, even if it's in their best interest. Chapter 16 provides a deeper discussion and other cases involving these basic medical ethical principles.

Even in an emergent situation, you should involve other team members in your decision- making. You should also consider consulting with the hospital's administration and legal team.

In general, when asked to respond to any questions that involve ethical principles, it's always important to demonstrate to interviewers that you would confer with others whenever possible.

One other important point: if you have any personal experience with such a situation, that can be helpful to add in.

Ways to Approach Blood Loss in a Jehovah's Witness Patient

Conscious and Coherent:

The first thing to do in this situation is to ask the patient. They can obviously tell you their wishes. You would proceed or not proceed with a blood transfusion depending on the patient's wishes.

Unconscious:

If a patient is unconscious, you may need to turn to collateral sources of information.

- You can look through the hospital record or chart, and see if there's any notation or documentation of the patient's wishes. Have they made a specific request not to be transfused in the past?

- Some Jehovah's Witness patients carry advanced directive cards with them, on their person, indicating their wishes regarding blood transfusions. Always look for any advance directives.

- If such information is not available, you can contact a relative or other loved ones. They can inform you what the patient would have wanted.

Unconscious and No Further Information is Available:

If you have no information about the patient's wishes, you are obliged to act in the patient's best interest. In the case of a bleeding patient, you would focus on stopping the bleeding. If blood transfusion is necessary then you may choose to do so. It's extremely important to document what happened and why you did what you did.

This action is in agreement with the Health Care Consent Act, which states that medical treatment may be given without consent in an emergency.

Once the patient is stabilized, you need to discuss the situation with the hospital administration as there are potential legal ramifications to your actions.

Case #9

While on a cruise, Mr. C developed flu-like symptoms. He felt too ill to go on a prepaid shore excursion. Upon returning home, he is informed by the travel company that the money spent for the excursion can only be refunded with a signed doctor's note. He asks his physician to write a note indicating that he was ill. How would you handle this situation if you were the physician?

Sample Answer

If I understand the situation correctly, the patient became ill while vacationing on a cruise ship. He had paid for a shore excursion. Because of his illness, he was unable to take part in the excursion, and now seeks a refund. The travel company has informed him that a refund can only be given if he has a signed doctor's note. He has asked his physician to write this note. Do you feel that I have a good understanding of the scenario?

Physicians are motivated to act in the best interests of their patients. Sometimes, they may be placed in positions in which they are called upon to deceive others. I would imagine that some situations would be more difficult to handle than others, especially if the patient stands to gain medical or social benefits. However, in this particular case, I believe that there are strong reasons not to write this note.

Lying and deception undermine social trust. If a physician lies, what reason would anyone have to believe him later? That's a real problem for physicians because the relationship between doctors, patients, and society depends on trust. Physicians have to routinely deal with third parties, and there is an expectation that the physician will be truthful.

In terms of how I would handle this situation if I were the physician, I would initially consider whether an important health benefit is at stake. In this case, health care isn't an issue. The patient wants a refund. Since it's not a medical issue, I don't think I have an obligation as a physician to help the patient.

Analysis

Note how the student provides a summary of the case. At the end, the interviewee asks if he has a solid grasp of the scenario. As physicians, we often do the same after we take a patient history. We check in with the patient to make sure we have an accurate understanding.

In the introduction, the student acknowledges the difficulty of the situation. Of note, he ends the introduction with a statement indicating his position. Now the interviewer will expect to hear the reasons why the interviewee feels this way.

Here the interviewee offers the reasoning behind the position he has taken.

Now the interviewee applies his thought process to the scenario, making sure to answer the question, "How would you handle this situation if you were the physician?"

Before I present my position to the patient, I would first inquire about the patient's health. How is he feeling? Is he over the flu-like illness? How did the rest of the trip go?

The interviewee shows concern for the patient, an important quality to demonstrate during the MMI.

After doing so, I would explain to the patient why I'm unable to write the note. I would remind the patient that I have two ethical duties – to help him and be truthful. If I mislead the travel company, how would my patients trust me not to mislead them in other situations? I would also point out problems that will occur if the travel agency makes further inquiries. This has ramifications for both the doctor and the patient.

After showing concern, he explains the approach he would take with the patient.

However, I would help the patient find other solutions. If the patient had seen the ship's doctor, I would encourage him to contact the cruise line to obtain the proper documentation. If the patient had not visited the doctor, perhaps the ship can still provide documentation that would be accepted by the travel company. Maybe the patient could speak with a manager at the company who might be able to award him credit for future travel.

Recognizing that this is something important to the patient, the interviewee continues to show concern for the patient by exploring other options.

In summary, although it would be unethical for me to write a note for this patient, I would do whatever I could to help the patient find another solution.

The interviewee closes with the summary statement.

Case #9: Key Points

- Patients seeking benefits frequently ask physicians to communicate with third parties. These parties include employers, schools, and insurance companies.
- At times, physicians may be tempted to deceive third parties in an effort to secure benefits for their patients.
- In one study, 39% of physicians reported one or more of the following tactics within the past year:
  - Exaggerating severity of patients' conditions
  - Changing billing diagnoses
  - Reporting signs or symptoms not present to secure patients coverage for needed care

---

To Deceive or Not Deceive...

Reasons for Deception

- Deception is in the best interests of the patient (e.g., "I did it because I felt that it was unfair for the insurance plan to deny a test which was necessary.")
- Benefits outweigh the harms

Reasons against Deception

- Deception is problematic because it undermines social trust.
- Harms outweigh benefits

Approach to Handling Deception Situations Involving Third Parties

- Step 1: Is there a health benefit at stake? If so, how important is the benefit?
- Step 2: Can the situation be resolved without deception?
- Step 3: Consider other options carefully.
- Step 4: Gently discuss the situation with the patient, including the consequences of deception for all parties involved, including patient, physician, and third party.

Similar MMI Scenarios

For the past month, a pediatrician has been evaluating a child for abdominal pain. Tests have been normal, and the cause of the abdominal pain is not yet clear. The parent calls the office asking for a note from the pediatrician. The child has not been able to participate in weekly swimming lessons because of the pain. The aquatics center will allow make-up classes if the parent is able to provide a doctor's note indicating that illness prevented the child from participating. Discuss how you would handle the situation if you were the pediatrician.

One of your patients asks you for a disabled parking permit. He does not have a medical indication for a permit. It turns out that his mother is visiting him from China. She has severe arthritis, and finds it difficult to walk long distances. He is hoping that you will sign the permit application so that he can take trips to the store more easily with her. Discuss how you would handle the situation.

References

Wynia M, Cummins D, VanGeest J, Wilson I. Physician manipulation of reimbursement rules for patients: Between a rock and a hard place. *JAMA* 2000; 283: 1858-65.

Case #10

Mr. J is a 62-year-old man who returns to his physician for a follow-up appointment. At the last appointment, he had reported upper abdominal pain and weight loss. Tests were ordered, and the results raised concern for possible cancer of the pancreas. The diagnosis can be established by needle biopsy. As the physician prepares to disclose the test results, the patient says, "The Missus and I are getting ready to take an Alaskan cruise. I sure hope that the news is good." The physician silently debates whether to delay this discussion until after the cruise. Should the physician inform the patient of his concerns about possible cancer?

Sample Answer

I can imagine that the patient and his wife have been really looking forward to this trip. From what I've heard, an Alaskan cruise is an amazing experience. I can see how the physician would be concerned that disclosing his fears about possible pancreatic cancer could affect the patient's travel plans, including cancellation of the trip. That said, I believe there are strong reasons for the physician to be truthful.

First, I believe that a physician has a strong moral duty to tell the truth since trust is at the heart of the doctor – patient relationship.

Second, the patient has to make some important decisions regarding diagnosis and treatment. He needs to know the truth so he can make informed decisions.

Third, if the physician conceals the truth, how will this affect their relationship moving forward? It seems as if the patient's life will change significantly, and it will be important for the patient to have confidence in the physician and their relationship.

Fourth, if physicians begin concealing the truth, then the public would lose faith in the medical profession. This could prevent people from seeking care when it's needed.

Finally, I would say that illness may not be convenient. The timing can never be predicted. Although the doctor may be uneasy about disclosing this information prior to the patient's cruise, there may never be a good time to have such a discussion.

Analysis

It is clear that the interviewee understands the physician's dilemma. He ends the introduction by taking a position. The interviewer will now expect to hear the reasons why the interviewee has chosen this position.

By using transition words ("First") between major points, the interviewee makes it easier for the interviewer to follow his line of reasoning.

In presenting your position, consider the consequences of your position with respect to all stakeholders. Here the interviewee addresses the potential impact on the public.

In summary, I would favor being truthful. This would allow both parties to discuss options for diagnosis and treatment. Although it may lead to a delay or even cancellation of the trip, it gives Mr. J an opportunity to make informed decisions.

Case #10: Key Points

- Honesty in all professional interactions is recommended by major organizations, such as the American Medical Association and United Kingdom's General Medical Council.

- Under certain circumstances, however, some physicians believe that deceiving patients is morally acceptable.

- There are no guidelines available to help physicians determine when deception is morally acceptable.

To Deceive or Not Deceive...

Reasons Why Physicians Deceive Patients

- Avoid physical or psychological harm to the patient
- Maintain hope
- Lessen stress or anxiety
- Patient does not wish to know the information
- Patient is unable to handle the information (emotionally or cognitively)
- Temporary deception to avoid great distress

Reasons Why Physicians Should Not Deceive Patients

- Violates physician code of ethics
- Patient will lose trust in physician
- Public will lose trust in physician and profession
- Emotional distress caused by discovery of deception
- Failure to respect or enhance patient's immediate autonomy
- Initial deception may lead to further deception

Sokol D. Can deceiving patients be morally acceptable? *BMJ* 2007; 334 (7601): 984-6.

Case #11

Ms. F is a 60-year-old woman who recently suffered a heart attack. After an extensive evaluation, her cardiologist has recommended bypass surgery to restore normal blood flow to the heart. The surgery has traditionally required the patient's breastbone to be split for access to the heart. A new technique, termed "mini" bypass, is now available and can be done by just making several smaller incisions. This technique causes less pain and is associated with a shorter recovery period. The cardiologist has referred Ms. F to a cardiothoracic surgeon who will perform the bypass surgery. This particular surgeon prefers traditional surgery over "mini" bypass, and does not perform the newer procedure. Should he even discuss "mini" bypass with Ms. F? Explain your reasoning.

Sample Answer

Having just had a heart attack, I imagine that this is a difficult time in this patient's life. Now her cardiologist, after evaluating her, has recommended bypass surgery. The cardiothoracic surgeon seems skilled in the traditional method of performing bypass. However, there is a new method that apparently has some benefits, which include less pain and shorter recovery time. Since the surgeon doesn't perform this new surgery, should he even discuss it with the patient? If I understand the situation, that's the central issue here. Do you feel that I have a good grasp of the case?

Before I address whether the surgeon should inform the patient about the new surgical approach, I will say that patients need to know the nature of any surgery planned, how it will benefit them, the associated risks, and alternatives to surgery. With this knowledge in hand, the patient can then make an informed decision about what she would like. That's the basis of informed consent, and the focus of this case.

In this case, it seems clear that surgery is needed. If the patient understands that and wishes to proceed with surgery, then a more detailed discussion about surgical approaches would seem reasonable. I realize that the surgeon doesn't perform the "mini" bypass but I do believe that it's important that he discuss this new technique with her.

If the patient knows that the new procedure is less painful and leads to faster recovery, then she may be more inclined to have it done in this manner. Not being told of this option would prevent her from making an

Analysis

Informed consent is legally required. Doctors have an obligation to inform patients who are deemed competent of the proposed plan. This includes surgery, test, procedure, or medication.

The applicant's position is very clear.

informed decision, and could lead to suboptimal care.

From the surgeon's perspective, he may have some concerns about the procedure. Perhaps he's concerned about outcomes. Maybe long-term data is lacking, and that's why he prefers the traditional approach. It may be that he's simply more comfortable with the traditional surgery. I think it would be okay to talk about these concerns, and the patient would probably welcome his perspective.

Always try to consider the other side of the argument.

If this new approach had no scientific basis or evidence to support it, then I could understand not bringing it up. But it seems like there is some research to back up this new technique, and I feel like other physicians in the field might recommend it.

If alternative treatment options have no scientific support and are not effective, the doctor does not need to mention these treatments.

In closing, I believe the surgeon should discuss both surgical approaches. My feeling is that the patient should have the right to choose among these feasible options. It's the physician's job to educate the patient and make recommendations. Only after that can the patient make an informed decision that's in accordance with her goals and values. Even if it leads her to have the surgery done by someone else, it still seems the right way to handle things.

Case #12

You are a third-year medical student rotating through your internal medicine clerkship. During rounds with the resident, you examine together a new patient with a lower leg infection. The resident takes the history and performs the exam while you observe.

Later during rounds with the attending physician, you are present while the resident discusses the new patient. You are surprised when he mentions the results of a groin exam because you did not observe the resident performing this part of the physical exam.

Describe how you would handle this situation.

Sample Answer:

Student: We have a situation where I am a third-year medical student rounding with a resident and during the presentation of our patient to our attending, I hear the resident say that he completed a groin test which I did not see him do. I'm being asked to talk about how I would handle the situation. Do you believe I have a good understanding of the situation?

Interviewer: Yes, you do.

Student: The issue at hand that I see here is the implication that something wrong has been done and I think that this has several implications. I think it's incredibly important that we, as care providers, maintain a certain level of honesty, transparency, and communication when providing patient care.

And so as a medical student, I would have to make sure as a member of the team that everyone on the team is keeping patient safety and the patient's care as their number one goal.

Having said that, I also recognize that the relationship I have with the resident and the attending is very delicate and also very important. Therefore, I can't jump to any conclusions. It's important not to assume anything even if I think I know what happened.

I think the resident is saying that he did something that he didn't do, but I can't know that for sure. It may be the case that the resident came back and did the test when I wasn't there. It could be that because of my inexperience the test was done, but I

Analysis:

The applicant recaps the scenario, seeking confirmation that his understanding is correct.

In this case, the applicant makes sure to include that this is an "implication". In responding, therefore, he is describing how he would handle a situation in which he is concerned that a resident may have misrepresented care, the operative word being "may".

The applicant makes it clear that patient safety is the most important consideration, but he is also careful to consider all perspectives

The applicant describes not only the issue, but key values in healthcare.

didn't see it because I didn't recognize what that looked like.

So that's the first thing. I can't jump to any conclusions or assumptions.

Assuming that patient safety isn't immediately in danger, after rounds are completed, I would ask the resident to step aside to a private place where we could have a confidential discussion. And in a non-accusatory way, I would simply ask. "I'm a little bit confused on something. Do you mind if we recap something about Mr. Smith's case?"

The resident would say "yes" and I would say "I noticed that we said that we performed a part of the exam, but I didn't really catch that part. Can you walk me through it?"

And from that discussion I should be able to quickly find out what happened. The resident might say "this is when I did it and this is how I did it." Or I might hear "Oh, you know that's just what we always say, that it's always the same result."

He makes sure to describe possible alternative explanations.

I would quickly understand if the resident did or did not in fact do the test.

Once I had clarification, I could then act on the information. This again speaks to the idea of patient safety being the number one guiding factor, but also being aware of the nature and importance of relationships with our colleagues.

It's important to be aware that these situations will come up and they will test us as care providers. It's not only important to be ready to navigate these challenging situations, but to also keep patient safety and care as our guiding light

He includes a strong conclusion statement.

In responding to challenging scenarios such as this one, it's important to

1.Read the scenario
2. Clearly identify the question
3. Plot out the structure of your response
4. Include a strong conclusion

What made this a strong response?

1. The applicant clearly highlights important values. "Patient safety is our guiding light."
2. He makes it clear that although patient safety is paramount, it's very important to avoid jumping to conclusions.
3. He is actively seeking alternative explanations, and is directly seeking more information from the resident. Although he is asking directly, he is using a non-accusatory framing.

Remember that when responding to every one of these challenging scenarios, that there is no correct response. The strongest responses are those that demonstrate patient care and safety as the primary concern, and that also showcase the applicant's mature, empathetic, professional responses to a situation.

Case #13

You are completing your rotation in family practice. Your preceptor is an elderly physician working in a community clinic. Your next patient is a 16-year-old young man who reports a chronic runny nose. The mother explains that her son is extremely bothered by this, especially during school because he constantly has to wipe his nose. You know that there are likely effective treatments for this condition, once a work up has been done and the cause has been established. Your preceptor, however, tells the mother that this is a common condition--it is probably due to allergies, but there are no treatments available.

Please explain how you would handle the situation.

Sample Answer:

In this case, a young man is suffering with a symptom that is causing him distress. It appears that there are effective treatments that would alleviate his symptoms, but the family practice physician has not discussed these treatments with the family. Have I understood the case correctly?

This is a difficult situation, because this young man is clearly suffering from his condition. It might not be causing pain, but it is interfering with his quality of life. Our main goal in healthcare is to care for the patient, so I would plan to do whatever I could to help him improve his symptoms.

At the same time, I would not want to interfere with the physician-patient relationship. In thinking over what to do, these would be my two main considerations. Therefore, I would not speak up during the patient encounter itself. However, as soon as my preceptor and I had free time, I would ask my preceptor.

If I had some free time during the day, I would try to learn more about these potential treatments. I'm not sure if the preceptor is just not aware of these treatments, or for some reason has decided not to utilize them, but I would try to gently find out. Then I would ask my preceptor if he thought X medication might be an option for this patient. It is possible that there is a medical reason that I'm not aware of as to why this treatment could not be used. If, however, my preceptor was just not aware of this treatment, I would hope that he would be

Analysis:

The student highlights that this young patient is experiencing a poorer quality of life because of his symptoms. He emphasizes the need to care for the patient. It's important to recognize that even "not serious" symptoms can be of serious concern to patients when it interferes with their quality of life.

He also recognizes and verbalizes the importance of the physician-patient relationship. He makes it clear that his response to this situation is focused on these two main considerations.

He is giving a clear description of his next actions. In these types of scenarios, it is important to respond to the prompt. In this case, the student is clearly describing "how he would handle the situation." He doesn't just describe several potential options for handling the situation. He states what he would do, and the actions he would take if the preceptor did not respond to his prompting. "If my preceptor was not open to learning... Then I would..."

open to learning more about X treatment. If he was, I would volunteer to contact the patient and his mother myself and explain the benefits and risks of the treatment.

If my preceptor was not open to learning about new potential treatments, then I would seek out the medical school faculty in charge of the rotation for their advice and suggestions. I would definitely not act on my own since my preceptor is the patient's physician and I would not want to interfere with the physician-patient relationship, but I would continue to seek guidance since my patient's well-being is my main concern.

He describes additional steps he would take if necessary.

His final statement is that "the patient's well-being is my main concern."

Chapter 16:

Discussion Questions

Case #1

There are a number of important discoveries in medicine, from antibiotics to vaccines to ventilators. What do you consider to be one of the greatest discoveries in medicine?

Sample Answer

So many discoveries in medicine have had a tremendous impact. And although it's hard for me to single out one as the most impactful, I would like to share one discovery that I find simply amazing. It's the use of oral rehydration solution, which has saved the lives of over 50 million children suffering from vomiting and diarrhea.

I learned so much about it during my international health trip to Kenya. I went to Kenya with a team of healthcare professionals. We worked side by side with Kenyan doctors in rural parts of the country. We had a wonderful opportunity to care for patients who have limited access to health care.

One of the Kenyan doctors had told me about oral rehydration therapy, and how much of a difference it had made in his country. Amazingly, as a child he too had benefited from the solution. That made me think about how this solution has transformed lives and families, and allowed children to become adults.

It's amazing to think what some of these adults have done for our world, whether it's by becoming a nurse, a doctor, a researcher, and so on. When you look at it that way, the impact is tremendous, not only in terms of the lives saved, but in terms of the contributions these survivors have made to the world. I know that diarrhea is still a major cause of death in children. And I hope that with my interest in global health, that I can be a part of the solution.

Analysis

In analyzing this answer, it is clear that the interviewee has a strong knowledge about diarrheal illness in children and the use of oral rehydration therapy. The answer states the impact of the discovery in terms of lives saved. He weaves in his own story and demonstrates that he has an interest in global health. He ends by indicating that he hopes to make a difference in this field down the road.

This answer does a great job of answering a challenging question while also revealing something specific about the applicant.

Case #1: Key Points

Medical school interviewers have an appreciation for the history of medicine. They like to see that future physicians have given some thought to the history of the profession and how it has developed.

Many medical school leaders believe that historical perspectives are an important part of the medical school curriculum. In a survey of US medical schools, almost 40% had formal lectures or seminars about the history of medicine.

History teaches us about disease and how our approach to disease and treatment has changed over time. This requires an understanding of social, economic, and political forces. History provides us with this context.

If you search the internet, you'll find rankings of the most important discoveries or inventions in medicine. These rankings differ considerably as to what is considered the most important discovery.

What does that mean for you as an applicant when answering this interview question?

That means that there really is no right answer. There are so many discoveries that have had tremendous impact, and it's impossible for people to agree on the most impactful. Therefore, the best way to answer this question is by choosing one discovery and then doing your research.

Use the information that you learn to develop a powerful answer: one that reveals the depth of your knowledge as well as something about you.

In my experience, the most common answers given by applicants have to do with the discovery of penicillin or the use of vaccines. There's nothing wrong with discussing penicillin or vaccines, but it can be hard to stand out when just about every applicant is using one of these two discoveries in their answer.

Fortunately, there are plenty of other important discoveries—and just a little background reading will uncover the fascinating stories behind these other discoveries.

Also, remember that a response that includes something about you or your experiences (in addition to the discovery) will make for a more powerful response.

The History of Oral Rehydration Solutions

Back in the 1970s, around the time that India and Pakistan were firmly entrenched in a war, monsoon season hit. With its heavy rains and ensuing floods, it led to a calamitous situation for thousands and thousands of refugees. These refugees were deprived of necessities and poured into medical camps seeking assistance.

The Government of India, the state government of West Bengal, and a number of nongovernmental organizations sought to provide assistance. These overwhelmed organizations were taxed even further when a cholera epidemic broke out. Although IV saline solutions were available, they weren't enough to provide for the enormous population. There was also a lack of trained volunteers to administer them. Within a few days, 30% of patients died, many being children.

This disaster deeply affected Dilip Mahalanabis, a member of the staff of the Johns Hopkins Center for Medical Research and Training in Calcutta. Mahalanabis was part of a team that had developed a new oral rehydration solution to replace the water and electrolytes that are lost through vomiting and diarrhea.

He was not the first to discover oral rehydration therapy, but the therapy up until that point had only been used in tertiary referral centers. Dilip felt that this therapy could make a difference during the cholera epidemic.

He and his team worked feverishly—measuring the ingredients, placing them in plastic bags, writing out instructions, sealing the bags with a hot iron, and then sending them urgently to the camps.

The packets were received at the camps, and healthy family members and staff had their patients drink large volumes of this solution.

The Results of Oral Rehydration Solutions Were Simply Amazing

Over eight weeks, there was a steep drop in mortality—from almost 30% to less than 1%.

However, oral rehydration solutions were not accepted right away. Dilip wrote a paper about the dramatic results. Unfortunately, his findings were met with skepticism. Leading experts in the field rejected it.

This miraculous medical development might have ended there, if not for a cholera expert from the World Health Organization named Damon Baruah. He agreed to see things for himself.

And when he went, he was absolutely stunned by what he saw.

What he saw was the successful treatment of cholera with just oral rehydration solution. He realized that oral rehydration treatment could completely change the way in which diarrhea was treated all over the world. In his mind, he imagined millions of children's lives being saved.

He returned to the World Health Organization and shared what he had seen. This led to the creation of the World Health Organization's Diarrheal Disease Control Program. Studies were also done that showed no clinically important differences in effectiveness between oral and IV fluid replacement in children with diarrhea.

The impact of this discovery was enormous.

In the 1980s, close to five million children under the age of five years died each year from diarrhea. Twenty years later, that figure had dropped to 1.8 million.

In poor countries, children can expect to have three episodes of diarrhea every year, which means they face a potentially life-threatening infection as often as every four months. With oral rehydration therapy, their risk falls tremendously.

In the last 25 years, more than 50 million lives of children have been saved with oral rehydration therapy.

Although there have been tremendous strides in the treatment of diarrhea, it still remains the second most common cause of death among poor children. With this cheap and easily prepared solution, the world has the power to prevent even more deaths due to diarrhea.

Case #2

You are working in the emergency department and two patients arrive to the hospital at the same time. Both are in need of a ventilator, but the hospital only has one. The first patient is a 50-year-old physician, and the second patient is a 22-year-old retailer worker. Both patients are doing similarly clinically. What type of criteria would you use to decide who receives the ventilator?

Sample Answer:

The first criteria I would consider is patient likelihood of survival. Since both patients are clinically doing similarly, it seems the prognosis for both patients would be similar, so other criteria would take preference. However, I would also consider comorbid conditions for the patients, such as if one of them has diabetes or heart disease, as these issues may affect prognosis.

Next, I would consider patient age. The 22-year-old patient is younger and has had less of an opportunity to live. The 50-year-old patient has lived 28 years longer. Moreover, the 22-year-old is more likely to live for a greater number of years than the 50-year-old, given general life expectancy.

Another criterion I could use is past contribution to society. As the 50-year-old is a physician, they have dedicated much of their life to saving others and are highly trained, and they may continue to take care of patients in the future.

Finally, I would consider whether these individuals have children or dependents. For instance, if one patient were to have young children dependent on them, this is important to take into account, as opposed to a patient with no or adult children.

If possible, I would also inquire into whether it is possible to borrow a ventilator from another hospital, or if there is another intervention that could benefit one of the patients or alternative options.

Analysis:

The student focuses on the question in the prompt. The question is not "what would you do?" Instead, the question is "what type of criteria would you use to decide?" This is a common mistake with this type of prompt.

The use of words such as "the first criteria" and "next" are helpful in following the progression of the response.

Overall, I would consider prognosis and likelihood of survival, age, contribution to society, and children.

A strong concluding statement that summarizes the criteria discussed is very helpful.

Case #2: Key Points

There are several ethical principles that are regularly used in allocation of scarce medical resources, and a number are incorporated into this response.

The first ethical principles this answer uses are the concepts of youngest first, prognosis, and number of life years saved. Younger individuals have not had the opportunity to live as long, and prioritizing younger individuals, patients with a better prognosis, or less comorbid conditions, may result in an objectively greater number of "life years saved," because these patients are more likely to live longer following recovery.

Another consideration is patient likelihood of survival. Although in this case the patients are doing similarly clinically, other scenarios may present patients with different likelihoods of survival. For example, a case may present a patient with a 50% chance of survival, as compared to a patient with a 25% chance of survival. This is also important to consider.

It is ethically acceptable to consider instrumental value, or future usefulness of an individual, in triage decisions. For example, some ethical guidelines may prioritize health care workers, because they save the lives of other people.

This response also considers children. It would be prudent to contemplate whether the death of a patient would leave orphaned children.

This response also considers alternatives, such as seeking assistance from another hospital or alternative interventions.

References:

[1] Persad G, Wertheimer A, Emanuel EJ. Principles for allocation of scarce medical interventions. *Lancet.* 2009;373(9661):423-431. doi:10.1016/S0140-6736(09)60137-9

Case #3

An attending physician is in the habit of introducing third-year medical students rotating with him in the hospital as "Doctor." Discuss the ethical issues raised by this practice.

Sample Answer

I believe there are strong reasons to be truthful in these introductions.

First, it's important that patients trust their doctors. If the doctor misrepresents who the student is, the patient may feel betrayed when he discovers the student's true status. I feel that patients might perceive this practice as deceptive.

Second, doctors have the responsibility to reveal pertinent information to patients. It would be important for the patient to know who is involved in their care, their precise roles, and their responsibilities. Knowing all this may very well have an impact on the patient's decision-making. For example, let's say the patient needs a procedure. It would be well within his rights to refuse to have the procedure done by a student, but he would only be able to express that sentiment if he knew the student's true status.

Third, there may be legal requirements for students to inform patients of their educational status. Even if there are no legal requirements, there may be policies that have been put in place by the state medical board, hospital, or medical school. It would be important to adhere to these rules.

In trying to understand this from the doctor's perspective, I wonder if he's concerned that the patient may not allow the student to participate in his care if he knows the student's status. Or perhaps he feels that learning opportunities will be compromised if he uses the term "medical student." Although I can understand these concerns, I don't believe that they override the importance of maintaining trust.

Analysis

The interviewee takes a position from the start.

Each point offered to support the position is introduced by number ("first"), making it easier for the interviewer to process the information.

An example is offered to provide more strength for the point.

In concluding the response, the interviewer tries to understand the perspective of the doctor before leaving the interviewer with his final thoughts. His last words remain consistent with the position taken at the beginning.

Challenge Question

You are the medical student working with this attending physician. After entering the patient's room, you are introduced as "Doctor." The attending physician decides that a knee aspiration is needed for diagnosis. This is a procedure in which a needle is inserted into the joint space, and fluid is removed for testing. You have only seen the procedure performed once, and now your attending physician would like you to perform the procedure. How do you proceed?

Case #4

At a party, a group of medical students lament the good old days of medicine in which doctors were wined and dined and sent on lavish trips at the expense of pharmaceutical companies. "I don't get it," said one student. "We should still be able to receive gifts from drug companies." Discuss reasons for and against accepting drug company gifts.

Sample Answer

Although I understand reasons why some may feel that it's acceptable to receive gifts, I believe there are compelling reasons why doctors should not accept gifts.

I'd like to start with reasons to accept gifts. I've heard that education courses and meetings are sometimes subsidized by drug companies. In these situations, an argument can be made that this practice provides an important educational benefit. In working in free health clinics, I've also seen how many patients can't afford medications. In these cases, medications received as gifts allow for the proper treatment of these patients' medical conditions.

Reasons to not accept gifts have to do with objectivity. If drug companies fund educational conferences, I would be concerned that this might influence speakers and their slides. The material presented may be slanted towards a medication produced by the drug company. I would even worry about low-cost items like pens and notepads because if it's in front of you, you may be tempted to prescribe that medication.

I would also worry about how gifts would be viewed by patients. If it affects the trust patients have in their physicians, then it's a significant problem. Patients need to be confident that their doctors' behavior and practices are not being influenced by drug companies.

I have read that physician organizations have been enacting strict policies on the ways in which physicians interact with pharmaceutical companies. I would be in favor of policies that place the patients' best interests above other factors. For these reasons, I would not favor accepting gifts.

Analysis

As the interviewee offers reasons to accept gifts, he is effectively able to incorporate what he has observed as a volunteer in free health clinics. If you have personal experience related to the MMI scenario, consider weaving it into your discussion. This has the potential to elevate the strength of your answer.

In 2003, drug companies spent over $25 billion dollars promoting their drugs. Money was used to give doctors gifts and sponsor informational lunches. Although many physicians don't believe that this affects their prescribing practices, research has shown that these interactions often do.

Case #5

Following the death of their 17-year-old daughter in a car accident, the parents donated her organs and received permission from the courts to remove and freeze their daughter's eggs. Their intent is to have the eggs fertilized with donated sperm. Discuss the ethical issues involved.

Sample Answer

My heart really goes out to the parents of this 17-year-old who was killed in a car accident. Donating her organs has the potential to benefit other patients, but removing and freezing her eggs for fertilization raises some important ethical concerns.

In this situation, I would imagine that the parents are distraught. By harvesting and the fertilizing the eggs with sperm, they might feel that the child born would be one way to keep the memory of their daughter alive.

I wonder if the daughter had expressed a desire to have children before her death. Even if she had, I wonder if she was mature enough to truly understand what it means to be a mother. Since she would be unable to provide consent, the doctors involved would have to rely on the parents to make suitable decisions on her behalf.

Then I realized that the bigger issue is that any child conceived from fertilization of her eggs will never know her mother. Would the daughter have wanted a child to be born after she passed away? If she did, would she have wanted her own parents to raise her child? And what impact would this have on the child years later when she fully understands how she came into this world?

I'm not sure there are any easy answers to these questions. However, I might be inclined to encourage families to wait until enough time passes before making these important decisions. With time, the emotions which are so raw initially may lessen to some extent and allow loved ones to make a sound choice.

Analysis

The interviewee begins by showing concern and compassion for the parents who have just lost their child.

Benefits to the parents are discussed. A useful approach with ethical scenarios is to consider the perspectives of all stakeholders.

Interviewee discusses the situation from the perspective of the deceased. Also raised are important issues related to informed consent.

Additional concerns from the perspective of the deceased are presented. The interviewee also considers what effect this may have on the child conceived.

Interviewee recognizes the difficult issues raised, and does not profess to have all the answers. She ends with a very mature response on how she might guide such families dealing with the loss of a loved one.

Case #6

In 2005, after having her feeding tube removed by court order, Terri Schiavo passed away at the age of 41. She had been in a coma for fifteen years. During the last seven years of her life, there was a fierce battle between her husband and parents. Referring to conversations he had with Terri, the husband indicated that she never wanted to be kept alive artificially. Terri's parents were skeptical of his claims and argued vehemently to keep her alive. They remained hopeful that she would recover despite the fact that doctors disagreed. Terri's parents appealed to the governor, state legislature, and even the President of the United States. However, the courts consistently backed her husband's right to let his wife die. Discuss the issues involved.

Sample Answer

I remember being in high school at the time when the Terri Schiavo case gripped our nation. My heart really goes out to both her husband and parents. I can't imagine what it must have been like for them to go through all of it. From my perspective, I believe that the case highlighted some very important issues about advanced directives and who should make medical decisions for family members when they're not in the position to do so.

If I remember correctly, she had no written advanced directives. Without a living will, it can be difficult to know for sure what someone would want in an end-of-life situation. The living will would also make clear who she would have wanted to speak for her on her behalf if she became incapacitated. Unfortunately, the lack of advanced directives led to considerable emotional distress for all those involved.

Had a living will been present indicating that she wanted her husband to make decisions on her behalf, it's possible that her parents would have respected her wishes. This would have prevented the battle in the courts that was waged for so many years.

In my own family, I know that the case spurred us to have a conversation that we may not have had otherwise. It led my parents to prepare their advance directives and have these crucial conversations with their doctors. I hope that one of the lasting legacies of this sad case is to foster greater public awareness of the importance of living wills.

Analysis

The interviewee recalls the case, remembers feeling affected by it, and shows her human side. She then reveals the issues she will discuss, readying the interviewer for what's to come.

She identifies the central issue. She goes on to discuss how the lack of advance directives led to the problems.

She offers her thoughts on what might have happened had Terri Schiavo documented her wishes.

Here the interviewee relates the case to her own life.

During my oncology shadowing experience, one of the things I learned was the importance of having end-of-life discussions early on. My physician preceptor told me that it's important that we speak to families about these issues well in advance of when these decisions must be made. That way, when the time does occur, the family will know that they are making a decision that is consistent with what their loved one wanted.

The interviewee very effectively relates the case back to her own experiences shadowing. In doing so, she clearly conveys exposure to the medical profession.

In summary, as distressing as this case was, there's so much that we can learn from the events. I know my family and I benefitted from it, and I do hope others did as well. In the future, I hope to be like my oncology preceptor—someone who handles these important conversations in a delicate manner.

She provides an effective close to her discussion, focusing on what she's learned from the case, and how it will shape her future.

Case #6: Key Points

- When a patient lacks the capacity to make personal health decisions, physicians rely on surrogates to do so.
- Be familiar with the legal hierarchy of surrogate decision-makers.
- At the top of this hierarchy are court-appointed guardians and surrogates selected by patients (health care proxy). The latter becomes official when the patient completes a form designating the person as the health care proxy, and then has the form witnessed and notarized.
- If there is no court-appointed guardian or health care proxy, then family members may serve as surrogates in the following order: spouse, adult child, parent, sibling, and other relative.
- Note that domestic partners in some states are considered on the same level as spouses.
- If there are no family members, a close friend may serve as a surrogate.
- If no one is available, then the physician can make decisions on behalf of the patient, preferably after consultation with other physicians or the hospital Ethics Committee.

Challenge Questions for Surrogate Decision Making

What if the patient is a minor?

If it is a non-emergent medical decision involving a minor, the physician must secure consent from the minor's parent or guardian. In some states, certain medical treatments may be offered to minors without parental permission. These include prescriptions for birth control, abortion, and treatment of sexually transmitted diseases. Before your MMI, become familiar with the laws in the state you will be visiting.

What if the patient's adult children are the decision-makers but they don't agree?

In these cases, consensus is preferred. Some states will allow physicians to rely on a majority decision or ask adult children to identify one person to be the key decision-maker.

What if the physician doesn't agree with the ethical or legal appropriateness of a surrogate's medical decision?

Hospitals often have an institutional ethics committee, and physicians can consult with these committees when there is dispute over treatment decisions. If an appropriate resolution still can't be reached, a judicial review may be requested.

Case #7

Family members and friends often ask physicians for medical opinions, prescriptions for medication, and other types of treatment. Discuss the ethical issues raised by such situations.

Sample Answer

I would expect that physicians are often asked to dispense medical advice and prescribe treatment outside of the office or hospital. Although I can see why physicians would do so, I believe that physicians should refrain from this practice with few exceptions.

To begin with, I'd like to offer some reasons why physicians might want to treat their family members or friends. Physicians are well-qualified to diagnose and treat, and it may be more convenient for them to do so. For family members, setting up an appointment, waiting for the appointment, and taking time off from work are all hassles. It can be less time consuming if they simply turn to the physician who is already in their life.

What would concern me most about physicians treating family members is whether the personal relationship could impact the care that the doctor delivers. For example, what if it's a touchy issue or problem? The physician may be reluctant to explore certain parts of the history or even perform aspects of the physical exam. The same could be said about patients. I would worry about the family member or friend's degree of comfort sharing information or allowing an examination.

In the hospital or office, the physician may not have any trouble setting limits on what he would be willing to do. With a family member or friend, would the doctor feel inclined to handle problems that fall outside the scope of his training or practice? If so, that would pose a danger to the patient.

Analysis

A very clear position has been taken by this interviewee. Now the interviewer will expect to hear her reasoning.

Before offering support for her position, she describes why physicians may be inclined to treat family and friends. It shows that she understands different perspectives.

According to AMA Code of Medical Ethics, self-treatment or treatment of non-patients, including family and friends, is not recommended because professional objectivity may be compromised.

Another concern has to do with the outcome of any recommendation or treatment. You would hope that nothing bad would come of it but what if something's missed or the patient doesn't do well. What repercussions would that have on their relationship?

An exception I would make is for emergencies or when medical care can't be easily accessed. In these situations, I believe it makes sense for the doctor to diagnose and treat a family member or friend.

One thing I'm not sure about is whether there are any state laws or licensing body guidelines regarding this practice. I would certainly consult with these authorities when making any recommendations.

This is an excellent point. Don't hesitate to consult with others who may know more than you. A good physician always recognizes his or her limitations.

In summary, I don't believe that physicians should help their family members or friends with medical issues unless it's an emergency situation. The physician may feel pressured to do so but with a gentle explanation, I believe that most people would understand.

Note that most states require physicians to maintain written records of treatment for non-patients.

Challenge Questions for Treatment of Friends and Family

You're at Disney World on vacation with your family. Shortly after arriving in Orlando, your cousin develops an upper respiratory tract infection with fits of coughing that she fears will keep her awake at night. She asks you to prescribe a narcotic cough syrup. How do you proceed?

Physicians should not prescribe controlled substances for non-patients. Many states and licensing boards are very clear on this point. "Except in emergencies, it is not appropriate for physicians to write prescriptions for controlled substances for themselves or immediate family members," writes the New Hampshire Board of Medicine.

You are at a high school reunion, and an old friend asks your advice about some numbness and tingling he's been having in his left thigh. How do you proceed?

It's common for acquaintances and friends to ask physicians for medical advice in social settings. In these situations, it's rare for a physician to have the detailed information required to provide specific advice. Many physicians would offer general information and then ask the friend or acquaintance to follow-up with his or her own physician. "Based on what you've told me, I would recommend talking with your physician about…" Some physicians would not feel comfortable offering any advice and would cite ethical or legal reasons for their inability to do so.

While driving through rural Montana, your friend develops urinary symptoms, and you suspect she has a bladder infection. You believe she would benefit from antibiotics. She recently lost her job and doesn't have medical insurance. Should you prescribe antibiotics for her?

If medical care can't be easily accessed, it would be reasonable for physicians to treat friends or family, especially if there is an emergent need for treatment.

Case #8

You are the head of a committee that has been tasked with developing policy to guide allocation of donated organs for transplant. Discuss the issues you will consider in developing this policy.

Sample Answer

There are many ethical issues related to the allocation of human organs. These issues have raised many questions. How can organs be allocated fairly? What are the medical criteria that should be used for allocation? Should non-medical criteria be factors in the decision-making? These are all valid questions, and we need to have a system in place for allocation because the demand for organs greatly exceeds supply. The system that's chosen should be a just system.

Medical need would be an important part of this system. I would say that those in greatest need would be patients who would die soon without transplantation. It would make sense to give these patients priority on the waiting list over those who are stable.

In terms of allocation criteria, I would favor criteria that are solely medical. However, I do realize that a person's psychosocial issues need to be considered. If someone's social situation would affect the outcome of transplantation, then would it be appropriate to transplant the organ into that individual? For example, if the patient was homeless, then he may not be able to adhere to treatment recommendations. But who's to say that the patient with social issues can't overcome these issues with the right support?

Time spent on the waiting list is also an issue to consider. Many people believe that those who have been waiting longer should receive higher priority if the level of medical urgency was the same.

Analysis

In the United States, the United Network for Organ Sharing (UNOS) suggests allocation criteria. Transplantation centers usually keep their own waitlist based on UNOS criteria.

Scoring systems have been developed to determine severity of illness. In selecting liver recipients, for example, doctors use the MELD system which yields a severity of illness score based on laboratory tests.

Some people maintain that social worth should be considered in organ allocation decisions. Opponents argue that it is difficult to measure social worth. How can anyone objectively assess potential contributions someone may make to society in the future?

Location is another consideration. When an organ becomes available, it may be better for people who live closest to receive priority. This would be especially important if the success of transplantation drops the longer we wait.

In summary, these are the major factors I would use to help me develop a fair system for allocation of organs for transplantation. Because this is such an emotionally charged topic, I would rely on a team of experts to help guide me. I would consult with all stakeholders to understand different perspectives and viewpoints. In the end, we could develop a system based on consensus but I don't believe that we would be able to please everyone. Although we may not be able to please everyone, I would want the system to be transparent so that the public doesn't lose faith in the importance of organ donation.

This is a strong conclusion because the applicant informs the interviewer that he won't make such an important decision on his own. He will consult with leaders in the field, and obtain opinions of all stakeholders. He is not afraid to seek input from others. He also realizes that no matter which system is adopted, there's likely to be criticism. He ends with a key point. If the public doesn't believe the system is fair, they may be less willing to donate organs.

Challenge Questions for Allocation of Organs for Transplantation

What do you think about age as a criterion?

Some argue that it makes more sense to transplant organs in younger individuals. They maintain that an 80-year old organ recipient is very likely to pass away soon even with a transplant. Contrast this with a 25-year old who has many years of life left.

Age as a consideration is taken even further by some who argue that the quality of life is very different for younger and older individuals. They feel that the younger recipient would have many more enjoyable years left. Opponents maintain that quality of life is very subjective, and you can't know for sure if a younger or older recipient will have better quality of life in the years they have left to live.

What if the patient is at fault for the disease that now requires transplantation?

Alcohol abuse is one example. Some people argue that potential recipients who are fully or partially to blame for their illness should not have priority over others who have suffered for no fault of their own. However, others maintain that there are genetic and environmental predispositions to alcoholism, and therefore it would be unfair to penalize alcoholic patients for something they can't fully control. In clinical practice, transplant teams will often require patients to show proof of abstinence for a period of time. This is not done to hold the patient accountable for his actions but because continued alcohol abuse increases the risk of a poor outcome following transplantation.

What if the patient is not a citizen?

Should citizenship be a criterion for transplant? Some people strongly believe that organ recipients should be citizens. However, we don't restrict noncitizens from donating organs for transplant. Noncitizens also follow the laws of our country, and pay taxes to federal and state governments just like citizens. Noncitizens also are eligible to receive other types of medical care, so why should organ transplantation be any different?

References

Abouna G. Ethical issues in organ and tissue transplantation. *Exp Clin Transplant* 2003; 1 (2): 125-38.

Caplan A. Bioethics of organ transplantation. *Cold Spring Harb Perspect Med* 2014; 4 (3).

Case #9

Alzheimer's disease is an incurable disease of the brain that destroys memory and thinking skills. It is a slow disease that progresses in stages. In its early stage, patients have no symptoms. In its next stage, there are mild symptoms which are often simply attributed to the aging process. Recently, researchers reported promising preliminary results of a blood test developed to detect patients with Alzheimer's disease at a very early point. Discuss the pros and cons of having such a test available.

Sample Answer

This case really resonates with me because I volunteered in a nursing home where many of the patients had Alzheimer's disease. I've seen up close what the disease does to a person, and the effect that it has on the family. I remember reading a bit about the disease, and I was surprised to see how many people have Alzheimer's. A blood test that could detect patients with Alzheimer's disease early would be an exciting development but also one that could cause some problems.

If there was a blood test which would allow early detection, it's possible that treatment could be started earlier. The hope would be that early treatment might slow down the progression of the disease.

Early detection would also allow patients to make important decisions about their future. Patients would be able to make decisions at a time when their neurological function was relatively intact. These decisions would include how they would want to be taken care of once the Alzheimer's disease became much more symptomatic. They could be very specific and leave no doubt about their choices regarding medical and financial decisions. For example, patients could indicate how aggressive they wanted their medical care to be. They could appoint someone to make medical decisions on their behalf if they weren't able to. They could make arrangements with their family about how they will be taken care of. Will they be in a nursing home? If so, which one?

There's another potential benefit of the test. If patients knew they had Alzheimer's disease early, they might start doing all the

Analysis

The interviewee begins with a personal story of his involvement with Alzheimer's disease patients in the nursing home.

Currently available Alzheimer's medications can help with the management of symptoms but do not offer cure or stop progression of the disease. Over time, these drugs lose effectiveness.

In a study of Alzheimer's disease patients having no advance directives upon initial presentation for cognitive evaluation, only 39% had initiated advanced care planning by 5 years of follow-up.

things that they had delayed. If they knew their time was limited, they could take trips, strengthen bonds, and even clear up any conflicts in their life.

In terms of problems with a test of this sort, I could see how someone might be impacted with an early diagnosis. The patient could become stressed, depressed, or even anxious. It may be hard for the patient to live life with this sense of doom.

An early diagnosis would also affect the patient's relationships with family, friends, and coworkers. Others may begin treating the patient differently, and that might embarrass the patient.

Another problem would have to do with the test itself. How accurate is it? If a person was falsely diagnosed with early Alzheimer's because of the blood test, it would be so devastating. It would essentially destroy someone's life for no reason.

In summary, there are risks and benefits to the use of a test for early detection of Alzheimer's disease. Continued dialogue about this will be necessary to develop policies to guide decision-making.

This interviewee could also have examined the issue from the standpoint of cost benefits associated with early diagnosis. Billions of dollars are spent every year for long-term care of Alzheimer's disease patients. A significant portion of this expense is taken care of by the government through Medicaid and Medicare programs. Early diagnosis and treatment could significantly reduce costs.

References

Garand L, Dew M, Lingler J, DeKosky S. Incidence and predictors of advance care planning among persons with cognitive impairment. *Am J Geriatr Psychiatry* 2011; 19 (8): 712-20.

Case #10

After returning from Sierra Leone where she had nursed Ebola
Virus patients, Kaci Hickox was placed in an isolation tent in
New Jersey. At the time, she had no symptoms of infection.
Critical of her forced isolation, she was driven to her
boyfriend's home in Maine four days later. The Governor of
Maine ordered her to quarantine, but she refused to comply with
the order. Medical science has shown that a person infected
with the Ebola Virus doesn't become infectious until the onset
of symptoms such as fever. Discuss the ethical issues involved.

Sample Answer

What makes the United States great is the freedom to choose how we live our lives. So I can see how a quarantine order would be difficult for people because of its impact on individual freedom.

However, we also have a responsibility to the community and the public. And that's what quarantine asks us to do—protect the health of the public. In this case, the government is asking the nurse to not put others at risk.

In terms of the appropriateness of the quarantine order, I would first look at the risk involved. We have to ask ourselves how likely we are to be harmed and how great will the harm be. In the Ebola Virus crisis, the harm is of great magnitude—serious illness or even death.

Although risk is an important consideration, understanding the science behind the virus and its transmission is crucial. From my understanding, unless people exhibit symptoms, they are not contagious. So if someone is without symptoms, there would be no reason to severely restrict their movements. I believe to quarantine someone when harm is unlikely would be unfair.

What I would consider doing is separating people at risk of acquiring Ebola Virus into different groups. One group could be those exposed but asymptomatic. Another group would be patients who are symptomatic but not yet known to have infection. It's the latter group that I would consider quarantining and testing for the virus.

Analysis

The interviewee begins by discussing the importance of individual freedom. Also presented is the responsibility that people have to protect the community.

In medicine, if possible, we like to make decisions based on the available evidence.

Here the interviewee offers a strategy to divide people into different risk groups.

However, before resorting to quarantine, I would talk with public health officials about less restrictive ways to handle the situation. What about having the person stay at home voluntarily and monitoring themselves for symptoms? If the person notices a rise in temperature, then he or she can seek medical attention and then enter isolation.

It's the responsibility of governors to make important decisions on behalf of their constituents, so I can understand their desire to move quickly to protect the public. Their intentions are good but I do believe that decisions have to be made based on science rather than fear.

In summary, I would not favor mandating an Ebola Virus quarantine for all people traveling to the United States from affected countries. I base this recommendation on the available science. However, I do believe that individuals at risk for infection have a responsibility to the public to not put others in harm's way.

The interviewee realizes that quarantine may be needed, but looks for less restrictive ways to protect the public while maintaining the person's autonomy. She does not hesitate to seek the help of others.

The interviewee looks at the issue from the perspective of the governor.

Ethical Issues Related to Ebola Virus

In 2015, perhaps no other infectious disease received as much attention as the Ebola Virus Disease.

From the vantage point of the COVID pandemic, notice the differences in responding to this case as opposed to responding to COVID. When considering the usefulness or need for travel bans and quarantines, it's important to be guided by science.

The considerations for a pathogen such as COVID are markedly different due to the virus' transmission by asymptomatic infected individuals.

Chapter 20 provides COVID-specific scenarios.

Further questions related to infectious diseases:

- Is it ethically appropriate for healthcare professionals to opt out of care of patients with Ebola Virus Disease?

- Should residents be allowed to participate in the care of suspected or confirmed Ebola Virus Disease patients?

- Should Americans infected with the Ebola Virus be airlifted out of Africa when others are not?

- Should Americans infected with Ebola Virus be given a highly experimental treatment?

- Should Africans infected with Ebola Virus be given a highly experimental treatment?

Case #11

Hospitals are expected to comply with a new law about pricing transparency, effective as of 2021. Because of this law, hospitals must publish their prices for 300 common procedures, such as the price for childbirth or a colonoscopy.

Discuss the issues and implications of this law.

Sample Answer

I remember hearing about this law in the news when it was passed, and how patient rights advocates were so happy about it.

I think the intent of the law is a very important one, but one major point is that we need to make sure that the law is working for the purposes that it's intended. In other words, we need to make sure that pricing information is easily accessible to patients. At the same time, it will be very important to study the implementation of the law and its effects. One major concern is that we need to make sure the law doesn't have unintended consequences, such as patients and hospitals prioritizing price over quality.

I've read multiple stories in the New York Times and other media outlets about individual patients who have received outrageously high medical bills. This is one extreme, where certain hospitals or healthcare systems charge extreme prices, and patients only find out about it after they receive a medical bill. I've also read about how many bankruptcies are due to high medical bills. With more patients having insurance that mandates high deductibles and high-cost sharing, it's more important than ever that patients are prepared for the price of their medical procedures.

From that standpoint, this law is a very important one. Our goal in healthcare is to care for our patients. Part of that care means limiting their financial side effects.

Beyond individual patients, we also need to think about the effects on employers, hospitals, and the nation. Since many employers provide healthcare insurance, it's

Analysis

In discussing the issues and implications of this law, the student begins with a strong positioning statement. She clearly lays out the main issues that she sees with the law.

She describes what she has read about this issue and makes it clear that she has some knowledge about the topic, introducing the information about high deductibles and high cost-sharing medical insurance.

also very helpful for them to have more knowledge about the price of healthcare. Because our nation spends so much on healthcare, efforts to reduce healthcare spending overall are important. The hope is that if hospitals must be transparent about their pricing, perhaps they will be less likely to charge extremely high prices.

Having said that, we need to make sure that we study the effects of this law. Healthcare quality must not suffer.

For patients, we need to educate them that cost is definitely not the most important thing about healthcare. While price is very easy to report, quality is harder to measure and report. Patients of course recognize that, and many may still be likely to choose healthcare based on their doctor's recommendation or the recommendations from their friends and family.

For hospitals, it's of course very important that they stay financially healthy. We know that the closure of a single rural hospital can affect thousands of patients' healthcare, so we need to study the effects on hospitals. One issue of concern is that we need to ensure that hospitals do not start cutting prices at the expense of healthcare quality, just to be able to say that they are the lowest price in town. Healthcare is not a commodity, and hospitals are not Walmart, so low prices should not be the only consideration.

This is where I think it's so important to measure outcomes. We need to study the effects of this law not only on healthcare spending but also healthcare quality.

Overall, I think this is a very important law and will help protect patients from sticker

She describes the impact of the law on other stakeholders. "Beyond individual patients, we also need to think about the effects on..." In discussing issues around a topic, it's important to consider the perspectives of all of those who will be affected.

She transitions here to discussing the other potential implications of this law.

shock and financial hardship. However, this law will only be helpful for patients if it is implemented well and if this information is easily available to patients and easy to understand. At the same time, it's very important to measure the effects of this law. Ultimately, we don't want the pendulum to swing from one extreme of outrageous prices to the other extreme of low prices at the expense of healthcare quality.

She ends with a strong concluding statement, stating that this is a very important law but laying out her concerns about potential negative effects of the law. Her last sentence is a very strong one, summarizing her major concerns in one sentence.

Centers for Medicare and Medicaid Services (CMS)

Beginning January 1, 2021, a new regulation was put into place by the Centers for Medicare and Medicaid Services (CMS). This regulation is centered on hospital price transparency. Every hospital in the United States as of this date is required to provide clear and accessible pricing information online. This information is required to be provided in two different ways.

- First, as a comprehensive machine-readable file that includes all items and services provided by the hospital.

- Second, as a display of shoppable services in a consumer-friendly format.

This list will cover 300 different services, such as childbirth care, x-rays, and joint replacement surgeries. Importantly, the hospital must also provide estimated minimum and maximum costs.

The agency states that this will make it easier for consumers to compare prices across hospitals and to be able to estimate the cost of their healthcare before going to the hospital. The CMS is planning to audit a sample of hospitals, and hospitals that do not comply may face civil monetary penalties.

Case #11: Key Points

If you're not familiar with the way hospital pricing traditionally works, this may be a surprise.

Why is it such a big deal that hospitals are required to publish their prices?

For decades, this information has been kept secret. Hospitals would negotiate with insurers for prices for different medical procedures and items, and those prices would vary from insurer to insurer. Patients would only know about these prices after they received a bill from the hospital.

Proponents of this rule believe that this will result in lower costs and better quality of care for patients. They make the argument that healthcare in America is a free market, and as such, consumers need to know the prices that they will be paying in this market.

Right now, consumers do not know the price of a certain service or procedure. Surprisingly, the physicians themselves typically don't know the price either. Although there may be a published price, that price is typically much higher than the negotiated prices with different insurers.

Prices also may vary significantly between different hospitals in the same community. One study found that the highest and lowest sticker prices nationwide for the same healthcare services differed by almost 300% on average.

In one example described by NPR, one man in Florida experienced wildly different prices for two abdominal CT scans. The first scan cost close to $300, while the second scan cost close to $9000.

Do these price differences matter? Absolutely, even for patients with insurance. In the case described by NPR, the patient had insurance, but after insurance paid their share, the patient still was responsible for over $3000.

One major concern with this new requirement is that healthcare quality may suffer. Critics are concerned that patients may choose a lower priced (and lower quality healthcare provider) to save costs.

Researchers have begun to study the effects of this rule, and this research will continue. One study looked at a random sample of hospitals and found that 83 (of 100 hospitals studied) were non-compliant with at least one major requirement of this rule. Only 30 hospitals reported discounted cash prices in a machine-readable file.

In another study, researchers evaluated the public websites of 20 honor roll hospitals and compared prices. They found that cash prices for an MRI ranged from $464 to over $6000. Prices for joint replacement surgery ranged from $22,000 to over $71,000.

References

Gondi S, Beckman AL, Ofoje AA, Hinkes P, McWilliams JM. Early Hospital Compliance With Federal Requirements for Price Transparency. *JAMA Internal Medicine*. Published online June 14, 2021. doi:10.1001/jamainternmed.2021.2531

Availability of Prices for Shoppable Services on Hospital Internet Sites. Accessed August 4, 2021. https://www.ajmc.com/view/availability-of-prices-for-shoppable-services-on-hospital-internet-sites

Hospital Price Transparency | CMS. Accessed August 4, 2021. https://www.cms.gov/hospital-price-transparency

A Florida man got 2 CT scans, one in an outpatient facility and another in an ED. The latter cost 33 times more. Accessed August 4, 2021. https://www.beckershospitalreview.com/finance/a-florida-man-got-2-ct-scans-one-in-an-outpatient-facility-and-another-in-an-ed-the-later-cost-33-times-more.html

Case #12

Burnout is becoming more prevalent across the medical profession. Discuss steps that you, on an individual level, will take to prevent burnout.

Sample Answer

Over the last two years, I've worked part time in a dermatology clinic, and my mentor Dr. Katta and I have talked about burnout prevention. It's also an area that was discussed in a course I took last semester, professionalism in medicine.

I've learned that burnout is becoming more prevalent in the medical profession, and that it has the potential to interfere with patient care as well as cause significant effects on physician well-being, so I believe it's important to be very proactive and to institute strategies early in my career to prevent burnout.

I think of this as involving three main areas.

The first area to think about focuses on what tools I can use to help me in my work and improve my accuracy and efficiency. For example, I've read research showing that electronic medical records have contributed to burnout because they have added to the length of time of the patient encounter. Therefore, I would approach EMR technology the way I do all digital tools: I would really try to learn how to maximize the benefits of this tool and to maximize my efficient use of this tool.

Next, I would focus on teamwork. One of my mentors once told me that it's important to recognize that physicians are the leaders of an entire team of healthcare professionals. It's important to make sure that each of us is working at the highest levels of our capabilities. That means that I would look at the clinic workflow and try to ensure that tasks were handled by the appropriate person. From answering patient messages to caring

Analysis

The student describes her experiences learning about burnout in the medical profession.

She structures her response well, highlighting three main areas.

She describes some of the research that she has read in this area.

In describing the importance of teamwork, she demonstrates that she has knowledge and awareness about workflow in a medical setting.

for patients, I would focus on how each member of the team can play an important part and have a clearly defined role, which will help with the overall quality and efficiency of patient care.

Finally, the third area I would focus on would be on bringing my best self to work. My mentor Dr. Katta once told me that our patients deserve to be cared for by a physician who is the best version of themselves. Just from working in the clinic, I have seen that patients can be frightened, upset, or experiencing a number of strong emotions. As a physician, it will be up to us to help them not only with their medical problem, but also with the emotions that they are experiencing.

Here she describes her experience from working in the clinic, and what she has seen of patient emotions.

That means that I'm going to focus on bringing my best self to work, and that means making sure that I have thought about and worked towards getting adequate sleep, exercise, and nutrition. I've also thought proactively about stress reduction techniques, especially given some of my stressful semesters as a premed student. I'm going to make sure I continue to deploy those. In my case, I really rely on time with friends and family, as well as yoga and running, to help me with stress management.

This is a strong response, demonstrating that she has thought proactively about wellness and stress reduction techniques.

From what I've learned, one of the most important aspects of burnout prevention is recognizing that any physician may be at risk, so thinking about the strategies proactively is something that I believe is very important.

This summary sentence indicates that she has thought proactively about burnout prevention strategies.

Case #12: Key Points

Multiple research studies have worked to identify risk factors for physician burnout. Although not all studies have agreed, in general it's hard to predict the risk of burnout based on demographic factors such as age, gender, or income. This means that any physician is considered at risk and should proactively be working to reduce the risk of burnout.

I call this "working towards sustainable success." What measures can you take to achieve success and sustain that success? This is an important question to start thinking about early in your medical career.

It's of course important to approach this issue from a systems-wide lens. There are organizational factors that are known to significantly increase the risk of physician burnout, and it's definitely important for medical organizations to work to mitigate these systemic factors.

Another approach to battling burnout is on an individual level, and this focuses on the actions that medical professionals can take to protect themselves.

Research has demonstrated that the use of strategies to reduce personal and occupational stress is associated with lower levels of burnout. That makes intuitive sense, but it's important to translate that knowledge into daily actions.

In research terms, "stress is significantly negatively correlated with the use of personal and occupational strategies for coping with it." In one study, respondents used a variety of strategies to reduce personal stress. Frequent strategies included eating nutritious foods and scheduling time for self and family. Other common strategies were used to help cope with stress on the job, such as appreciating relationships with patients and participating in continuing medical education.

Physicians Who Are Able to Sustain Success Are Those Who Have Worked on this Issue from Multiple Angles.

- **Reducing occupational stress.** Dr. Dike Drummond has written about his five-part electronic medical record strategy. He's also written about ways to improve the efficiency of medical practice. These are great strategies to focus on occupational stress.
- **Reducing personal stress.** A number of resources detail practical strategies for reducing stress in the home and in personal relationships.
- **Learning to manage the inevitable stress that will occur in our lives.** It's important to think about stress management. This absolutely starts with stress reduction (incorporating strategies at work and at home that can reduce levels of stress), but stress management recognizes that each and every one of us will deal with stress in our lives. How do we respond to that stress when it arrives?

There's a lot of literature on healthy coping strategies, and it's important to start testing out these strategies before you really need them. Research has supported the use of mindfulness practices, physical exercise, high-quality sleep, social support, and high-quality nutrition. In fact, integrative psychiatry now recognizes the importance of lifestyle interventions in the treatment of depression and anxiety.

Ultimately, one of the most important aspects of burnout prevention is recognizing that each and every one of us is at risk, and to start thinking now about ways to mitigate that risk.

References

Lee FJ, Stewart M, Brown JB. Stress, burnout, and strategies for reducing them. *Can Fam Physician*. 2008;54(2):234-235.

Drummond D. Part II: Prevent Physician Burnout: 8 Ways to Lower Practice Stress and Get Home Sooner. *Mo Med*. 2016;113(5):332-335.

Know the signs of job burnout. Mayo Clinic. Accessed August 6, 2021. https://www.mayoclinic.org/healthy-lifestyle/adult-health/in-depth/burnout/art-20046642

Case #13

There has been a national reckoning on racism and its effects on almost every facet of our society. How does racism affect healthcare?

Sample Answer

It has been a challenging year in so many ways, but one thing that the tragedies of this last year have led to is an awareness of how racism impacts so many areas in our society. In terms of healthcare, I think about three major ways in which racism has significant impacts. This includes effects on multiple social determinants of health, the impact of implicit bias, and the diversity of our healthcare workforce.

One of the most eye-opening classes I took in college was a class on professionalism in medicine. During this class, we learned about the extensive body of research on social determinants of health. Racism can affect an individual's employment opportunities, housing opportunities, and even access to healthy food. All of these are social determinants of health, and so can directly play a role in an individual's health outcomes.

Implicit bias can also affect health outcomes. I read one study in which the researchers compared how often Caucasian patients were prescribed pain medication as compared to African American patients. They found that Caucasian patients were more likely to receive pain medication prescriptions, and the authors felt that this was due to implicit bias. The healthcare providers were not necessarily overtly racist, but it was hypothesized that they had preconceived notions about African American patients perhaps exhibiting more drug-seeking behavior. This is an area that definitely needs further study, because it can be hard to identify the effects of implicit bias.

Analysis

The student provides a clear structure to her response. Although there are many areas that she could focus on, she chooses to focus on three main areas, which provides a more coherent response.

Social determinants of health are key drivers of health outcomes.

The student highlights some of her reading on this topic.

Finally, racism can affect the makeup of our physician workforce. This may be due to multiple factors, such as a lack of educational opportunities, a lack of mentoring opportunities, and other factors. This relative lack of underrepresented minorities as healthcare providers can have effects on health outcomes. I know that a number of studies have shown that, broadly speaking, some patients may have better health outcomes when they are treated by physicians of the same race. It's thought that this may be because patients are more likely to trust and follow the advice of physicians who are of their same race.

Research in this area has demonstrated that a lack of representation among the physician workforce has led to documented impacts on health outcomes.

There are multiple other ways in which racism can affect healthcare, and there are a lot of nuances to this area, but I believe that these are three major areas that can affect health care and health outcomes, and these are areas that we need to study further and work to improve.

Case #13 Key Points:

The effect of racism on healthcare is a very broad and complex topic. In discussing this topic, it's important to keep your response focused. In preparing for this topic, it's important to read widely.

There are a number of important research studies that have worked to document the effects of racism in healthcare. There are also a number of areas in which further research is needed, in terms of both the effects of racism in healthcare as well as recommendations to combat these effects.

First, it's important to learn key definitions.

Key Definitions

Social determinants of health. These are defined as the conditions in the environments where people are born, live, learn, work, and age that ultimately affect a wide range of health and quality of life outcomes. (More information and data on SDOH is available on health.gov.) These have been divided into five main domains.

- Economic stability
- Education access and quality
- Healthcare access and quality
- Neighborhood and built environment
- Social and community context

Structural racism. This is also called systemic racism. "This is the normalizing and legitimizing of historical, cultural, institutional, and interpersonal dynamics that routinely advantage white people while producing cumulative and chronic adverse outcomes for people of color."

Institutional racism. These are the policies and practices within an institution that produce outcomes that over the long term favor a particular racial group. Institutional racism may be intentional or unintentional.

Individual racism. This includes both conscious and unconscious attitudes and behaviors that contribute to racism.

Anti-racism. This is the process of actively identifying and eliminating racism. This encompasses working on systems, policies, and attitudes.

Explicit bias. This refers to our conscious attitudes and beliefs about a group.

Implicit bias. These are unconscious attitudes and stereotypes that can manifest in the workplace, school setting, healthcare, and other areas. These can be difficult to combat because we are often unaware of our own unconscious biases. Our culture, upbringing, and media messaging all contribute to implicit bias.

In the United States, racism has unfortunately led to many long-term impacts. Generations have been impacted by inequities in access to education, employment opportunities, housing, and healthcare. These social determinants of health directly impact health outcomes. They are also closely intertwined. If a community lacks access to quality education, it affects employment opportunities. This limits access to the type of well-paying jobs that provide healthcare insurance as part of an employment benefits package.

Ultimately, the impacts of racism in our society are complex and significant. Addressing the impact of racism on healthcare is similarly complex and of significant importance.

In an editorial in the New England Journal of Medicine, the authors discussed diagnosing and treating systemic racism. They highlight some of the research in this area, including one randomized controlled trial that found that black men who were assigned to black physicians sought more preventive care than those assigned to a physician of a different race. This has important implications, especially in terms of reducing the cardiovascular mortality gap between black and white patients.

The authors also discussed several areas to work on. One involved increasing the numbers of black people in the medical workforce. Another involved the need for individuals to become more conscious of our biases when caring for minority patients. It is also important to acknowledge past injustices and listen and openly discuss racism and its health effects in conferences and the medical school curricula. For our students and trainees, it is important to provide training on cultural sensitivity and upstander training, as they should be trained in advocacy tools that can help their patients and colleagues.

What are organizations working on to improve the current situation?

The American Medical Association's House of Delegates voted to adopt guidelines addressing systemic racism in medicine. They recommend that healthcare organizations and systems use these guidelines to establish institutional policies. They recommend specific workplace policies that clearly define discrimination and systemic racism, as well as explicit and implicit bias. They recommend the establishment of training requirements in these areas and prioritize safety in reporting actions related to racism.

The Essential Hospitals Institute has published an informational brief that clearly outlines some of the impacts of racism on patients, on providers, and on the community, and then describes hospital strategies that can be used to combat structural racism.

These strategies include (among many others):

- Creating a positive culture. This includes publicly committing to combating structural racism, partnering with community organizations, and gathering data to identify and combat racism.
- Policies, programs, and initiatives. This includes institutional policies that support diversity in hiring and promotion, as well as providing training and mentoring to promote career advancement. It also includes empowering staff to educate other staff members.
- Investing in underrepresented groups to overcome systemic economic disadvantages. This may include buying locally or relocating headquarters to an economically disadvantaged area of their city.
- Enhancing clinical processes to reduce disparities. This includes efforts to improve access to and quality of care, such as funding mobile units to combat issues with patient transportation.

References

AMA adopts guidelines that confront systemic racism in medicine. American Medical Association. Accessed August 13, 2021. https://www.ama-assn.org/press-center/press-releases/ama-adopts-guidelines-confront-systemic-racism-medicine

Evans MK, Rosenbaum L, Malina D, Morrissey S, Rubin EJ. Diagnosing and Treating Systemic Racism. *New England Journal of Medicine*. 2020;383(3):274-276. doi:10.1056/NEJMe2021693

Social Determinants of Health - Healthy People 2030 | health.gov. Accessed August 13, 2021. https://health.gov/healthypeople/objectives-and-data/social-determinants-health

The Role of Essential Hospitals in Combating Structural Racism. Accessed August 12, 2021. https://essentialhospitals.org/wp-content/uploads/2020/10/StructuralRacismBrief-Oct2020.pdf

Chapter 17:

Discussion Questions:
Basic Medical Ethics

Introduction

In this chapter, we'll review some basic ethical cases. These can be very challenging cases, and it's important that physicians understand the basic underlying ethical principles of issues they may confront in practice.

The cases in this chapter cover several major issues, including:

- Patient privacy
- Situations in which you may need to breach patient confidentiality
- The balance between patient autonomy vs. beneficence
- Advance directives and living wills
- The importance of determining the patient's last known wishes
- What procedures a DNR [do not resuscitate] order covers

Four Major Ethical Principles

Before we present these cases, it's important that you know the four major ethical principles that apply to medicine.

Autonomy	Autonomy is one of the most important concepts to fully understand when it comes to applying medical ethics to patient care. Patient privacy can be considered a subset of patient autonomy. Essentially, patient autonomy is the principle that states patients get to decide what happens to their body. Autonomy is applicable to adult patients with the capacity to understand and make decisions.
Beneficence	As physicians, our job is to help our patients. That's the basic explanation of beneficence: a doctor must act in the patient's best interest.
Nonmaleficence	This is the principle of "first, do no harm."
Justice	Health care should be fair. Justice is about making our healthcare system fair and distributing medical resources in a fair manner.

I think we all understand how important each of these principles is, but medical ethics can be challenging because sometimes these principles directly contradict each other. In such cases, one principle may take precedence over another. For example, in many cases, patient autonomy will supersede the principles of beneficence and nonmaleficence.

Case #1

You are working in the emergency room and are treating a woman who has developed symptoms of a sexually transmitted disease. Upon testing, it is found that she has contracted syphilis. She pleads with you not to tell her husband about her diagnosis. What would you do?

Sample Answer

This is a challenging case, because although we need to protect patient privacy, we also have an obligation in certain situations to protect the health of others. Sometimes this is required by law, such as in cases of certain transmissible diseases. This includes certain sexually transmitted diseases and certain transmissible respiratory diseases such as tuberculosis. Syphilis falls into this category of diseases that must be reported to the health department.

In this case, I would speak to the patient further. I would explain that we were going to focus on treating her infection, but we are legally required to inform the health department, who would then be reaching out to her spouse. I would then ask about her concerns. Could we arrange for a meeting with a social worker, who could connect her to community resources if she needed any help? Was she concerned for her physical safety?

In terms of her medical care, we would do further testing for other sexually transmitted diseases, and I would make sure that she had a follow-up scheduled with her primary care physician. If she did not currently have one, I would do my best to help her arrange that.

In treating her, I would make sure that she felt safe and that she understood that we would support her.

Analysis

She clearly lays out the main ethical concerns in this case.

Although we have a legal obligation, our first concern is patient care. It's important to ask the patient about her concerns and provide resources. It's important to learn more about why the patient is pleading with you. Is she concerned for her safety?

It is also important to think about the implications of a diagnosis of a sexually transmitted disease. This patient may be at risk for other conditions.

This summary sentence focuses on patient care: making sure that the patient felt safe.

Case #1: Key Points

This case focuses on issues of patient privacy, but it also touches upon the need in our society to balance between personal privacy and public good.

Privacy is considered a subset of patient autonomy. Ethically and legally, patients get to decide not only what medical procedures are done to them, but also what kind of information is shared with others.

Patient privacy is also a significant legal concern for physicians. I still remember when the Health Information Portability and Accountability Act (HIPAA) was passed. Passage of this act meant that legal consequences would occur if those who had access to protected patient health information did not keep this information confidential. Information protected by HIPAA includes:

- Details about a patient's case
- The patient's diagnosis
- Test results
- Planned treatments

The general rule of HIPAA is that patient health information can only be shared with others if the patient has explicitly given permission for that release of information—ideally, in writing.

As an example, if this patient's husband were to call your office and request the test results that you performed last week, could you release that information, given that this is the patient's spouse?

The correct answer is no. You could not release that information, even to a spouse, unless your patient had provided permission to do so and you had documented that in the chart.

The bottom line is that patients have a right to privacy. If you are going to breach that patient privacy (aka breach patient confidentiality), you must have a good reason.

When It Is Permissible to Breach Patient Confidentiality

The general rule of thumb is that it is permissible to breach patient confidentiality when it serves the public good. Certain diagnoses pose a risk to the public, and therefore must be disclosed.

Therefore, certain diagnoses are reportable to the local health department even without the patient's permission. These include:

- Certain sexually transmitted diseases, including syphilis
- Certain airborne respiratory diseases, such as tuberculosis

It is considered in the public good to know about these types of transmissible diseases, and you are therefore legally and ethically able to breach confidentiality in these cases. The health department would then act to notify the patient's contacts who are at risk.

- There are other instances in which you are required to breach patient confidentiality, such as when there is an immediate and documented threat to public safety. This may arise, for example, if a patient expresses homicidal thoughts during therapy.

Case #2

You are an Internal Medicine physician. Your next patient is a 45-year-old mother of two who comes in because she has felt a breast lump. You palpate the lump and because of your concern for breast cancer, you recommend that she get a mammogram this week.

However, the patient refuses. According to her religious beliefs, if this was cancer, she would not undergo treatment. You speak to her at length. You determine that she is rational and understands the potential consequences of not getting further testing.

What do you do next?

Sample Answer

Given my concern for breast cancer, this is a very challenging situation. I want to do what's best for the patient, but I also need to honor her religious beliefs. Therefore, I would try to explore her beliefs further and try to determine the specifics of those beliefs. It may be that this is not actually an "all or nothing" situation, meaning this may not be a situation where we have to either do nothing at all or do everything.

Therefore, I would ask her to return for a follow-up visit so we could discuss potential next steps. I would ask her if she would like to return with her spouse or a family member for additional support as I explain the potential outcomes of testing versus not testing. I would also ask if it would be possible to involve her religious counselor. I would like to explore further to see if there are any other treatment options available. For example, are there any treatment options that would honor her belief system? For example, perhaps she is not able to undergo surgery or chemotherapy but would be able to undergo radiation therapy. I would also ask her more about the benefits of diagnosis. Even if no treatment options at all were possible, would a diagnosis allow her to better prepare her family?

I would focus my efforts on honoring her wishes regarding her medical care, but I would explore much more deeply the extent of her religious beliefs and what these would allow in terms of diagnosis and treatment.

Analysis

Many ethical situations in medicine are not "all or nothing" situations. Exploring a patient's beliefs is a strong first step here.

The student does a good job of considering multiple different ways to explore the patient's beliefs further, while providing her additional social support.

The student also considers how the patient's beliefs might impact her treatment options. It is important to consider multiple different treatment options, as some may honor the patient's religious beliefs while still providing good medical outcomes.

This concluding sentence summarizes the student's response well.

Case #2: Key Points

The key ethical principle underlying your response here is autonomy, and this is an important one. As doctors, our key driving principle is often beneficence (helping our patient). However, patient autonomy generally takes precedence over beneficence. In this case, there are two key features:

- The patient is an adult
- The patient has the capacity to understand the consequences of not getting further testing

The principle of autonomy states that if you have an adult patient who has the capacity to understand, then the patient gets to decide what happens to their body.

However, it's important to remember that most real-life cases are rarely "all or nothing." As in your response, it's important to explore the specifics of the patient's belief system further and to involve family members and religious counselors with the patient's permission.

Case #3

(Note: This case is included to demonstrate several key basic points in medical ethics. This is a teaching case and not a typical MMI scenario.)

Your 45-year-old patient had originally declined a mammogram due to her religious beliefs (she does not believe in cancer treatment.) You successfully arranged a follow-up appointment with the patient and her husband, and had received the input of their religious counselor. The patient had decided that she would get a mammogram and breast biopsy if needed. If the biopsy showed breast cancer, she would proceed with radiation therapy, but would not use chemotherapy.

In order to make her wishes legally binding in case she became incapacitated in any way, the patient completed an advance directive in the form of a living will. In this document, she stated those wishes. In her living will, she specifically stated that she would not want surgery of any type for any reason.

Unfortunately, the patient was in a car accident and was brought to the emergency room with a broken arm. In the ER, you explain to her that although there's a chance that the arm will heal with just a cast alone, the orthopedic surgeon is recommending surgery for the best chance of proper healing.

After an explanation of the potential benefits, the risks, and the alternatives, she agrees to proceed. She explains that she understands what you have explained and would like the surgery. However, she then loses consciousness. When her husband arrives in the emergency room, he declines the surgery. He states that she has clearly indicated in her living will and to himself that she does not want any surgical procedures of any type for any reason. What do you do?

Sample Answer

Although this is causing concern to the husband, I would explain to him that the patient expressed her wishes to me directly before she lost consciousness, and she understood the benefits and risks of the surgery. Therefore, we would be proceeding with the surgical procedure. Although she has a living will, we must abide by her last known wishes.

Analysis

This case is included to demonstrate several key points. Although the response is short and to the point, it's important to recognize these key points.

Case #3: Key Points

This is a very long case description, but it's an important example of several key principles and practices such as patient autonomy, the use of advance directives, and the importance of the patient's last known wishes.

This case centers on the key principle of patient autonomy. In cases like this, honoring the patient's autonomy comes down to understanding their last known wishes. I call this the principle of "following the patient's last known wishes."

Although the patient has an advance directive in the form of a living will, she is able to make her wishes known in the ER. Therefore, her last known wishes are to proceed with the surgery. Importantly, the question made it clear that she had the capacity to understand this decision.

Follow this progression to honor the patient's last known wishes:

1. Follow a patient's last known expressed wishes, assuming she had the capacity to understand.

2. If the patient's last known wishes are unknown, then adhere to the preferences specified in their living will.

3. A living will is one type of advance directive. Advance directives are used when the patient becomes incapacitated. However, the wishes of a patient with capacity always take precedence.

4. If there are no advance directives available (or if the ones that are available don't cover this particular situation), then you would turn to a family member or loved one who is clearly familiar with what the patient would want.

5. This is a gray area, but if there is documentation of some type available, it can be used to indicate the patient's last known wishes. An example would be a letter written to a friend.

6. If there is no documentation of what the patient would have wanted, then you turn to the family for assistance in medical decision-making. Specifically, you would turn to the spouse first, then to adult children, then to parents, then siblings.

Documents That Support a Patient's Autonomy	
Advance Directives	These are very important documents, and it's important to understand what they are and how they are used. As the name suggests, advance directives are made in advance, and they direct the physician. These are legal documents that are filed in advance by the patient, and they specifically list the patient's wishes for health care in case the patient ever becomes incapacitated.
Living Will	This is one type of advance directive. A living will might state, for example, that a patient would never wish to receive a feeding tube or dialysis if she were to become incapacitated. Living wills may state as much or as little detail as a patient wishes, but the best ones are detailed and robust documents.
DNR Orders	This is one type of advance directive. There are frequent misconceptions about DNR orders. DNR stands for "do not resuscitate." Therefore, these orders only apply in cases where the patient has died. In other words, these only apply to measures such as CPR or defibrillation. These orders do not apply to surgery, cardiac catheterization, invasive procedures, dialysis, or other medical procedures.
Durable Power of Attorney for Healthcare	This is one type of advance directive. With this document, a patient would identify another person who will make decisions for her in case she were to become incapacitated.

In discussing advance directives, it's clear that many patients hold a number of misconceptions about these important legal documents. Politicians sometimes take advantage of this confusion to make it sound as though advance directives are the type of documents that would allow a doctor to "pull the plug" on a beloved family member.

Nothing could be further from the truth.

Because of these misconceptions, it's very important that all healthcare professionals educate our patients on the truth about advance directives. These documents outline a patient's wishes for medical care. The key is that the patient gets to decide.

These are really important documents for patients who have terminal illnesses such as metastatic cancer, or even those who are at high risk for sudden death, such as those with severe cardiac disease. However, advance directives can be created by any patient and can provide a strong sense of relief that a patient's wishes regarding their medical care will be honored, even if they cannot express those wishes at the time of medical care.

Case #4

(Note: This case is included as a teaching case, not as a typical MMI scenario.)

Your patient is a 60-year-old woman who is married and has two adult children. She presents with a breast mass. The following week, while she is awaiting her breast biopsy, she develops a stroke and becomes incapacitated.

Evaluation reveals breast cancer metastatic to the brain. One of the children states that her mom told her that she would never want a feeding tube, but the patient's husband and other child disagree. There are no advance directives or other documentation of the patient's wishes available. What would you do?

Sample Answer

This is a very sad case, and it highlights how helpful an advance directive would have been. Unfortunately, it appears that we do not have agreement on the patient's wishes. As the physician, she had not made her wishes clear to me. One child states that she knows what her mother wants, but this child doesn't have any documentation.

Therefore, I would consult the Ethics Committee. They will arrange a meeting and help facilitate open communication between the healthcare team and the family members. We would discuss the patient's prognosis, the possible treatments to help keep her as comfortable as possible, and try to get a deeper understanding of what the patient would have wanted.

Analysis

This is a helpful summary of the main issue in this case.

Ethics committees play a very important role in hospitals today. As medicine increases in complexity, it is important to have avenues for open communication between different family members, different physicians on the same healthcare team, and between physicians and family members.

Case #4: Key Points

Ethics Committees don't issue binding legal judgments. Instead, their goal is to facilitate open communication and to advise providers and patients and families about making healthcare choices while keeping what's best for the patient at the center of their discussion. They're often consulted when the doctor and the patient disagree, or when different doctors disagree about the best course of treatment. They're also consulted when family members disagree about the course of treatment.

These committees are usually composed of some combination of doctors, nurses, administrators, social workers, lawyers, and clergy. Sometimes these committees include laypeople.

Case #5

You are a pediatrician, and you are examining your 16-year-old patient during her annual well-child exam. She asks you for an HIV test but does not want her parents to know. What would you do?

Sample Answer:

In this case, I would explain to the patient that I can order the test without notifying her parents, but it's very important that we discuss her reasons for requesting this test first. If she is sexually active, does she understand how to protect herself against sexually transmitted diseases? If she is sexually active in the context of a relationship, does she understand how to have a safe and mutually respectful relationship? If she is sexually active and not in a relationship, is that by her choice?

Especially in the case of an adolescent who may be keeping certain behaviors from her parents, I would first want to understand why that is the case, and make sure she is safe and protected.

After that, I would encourage her to speak to her parents if she felt safe doing so. Regardless, I would explain that our visit would remain confidential and that I was available to her if she had further questions or concerns.

Finally, I would order the HIV test, as minors in the United States can legally obtain testing for sexually transmitted diseases without requiring parental notification.

Analysis:

Legally, the physician may proceed with the test, but the student here demonstrates that it is important to consider all of the ramifications of an adolescent who is seeking testing for a sexually transmitted disease.

The student recognizes the importance of the child parent relationship. She also makes it clear that she is available to the patient for further concerns.

The concluding statement focuses on the legality of ordering the testing.

Case #5: Key Points

Adolescent medicine presents unique challenges. One of these is that a patient who is a minor may wish to keep aspects of their medical care private from their parents.

This brings up medical, ethical, and legal concerns.

Medically and ethically, as physicians we are focused on the health of our patient. This includes understanding our patient's current knowledge and awareness of risk factors. Preventive medicine is important, and that means eliciting a complete and accurate medical and social history.

In the case of a patient who is a minor, patient education becomes even more important. How much does our patient understand about risk factors for sexually transmitted diseases? We must also ensure the safety of our patient, and questions on relationships are important.

Issues of Autonomy in Minors

The general rule is that minors do not get to decide what medical care is provided.

Remember, autonomy is defined as an adult patient with capacity. In general, minors don't get to decide their medical care; their parents get to decide their medical care.

However, there are exceptions, and it's important to learn these exceptions.

When can minors decide for themselves what's done to their body? In all states, minors can obtain testing for sexually transmitted diseases. In this case, you could order the HIV test without any concerns.

Regulations That Vary from State to State:

- In many states, minors can seek treatment for substance abuse without parental notification or permission.

- In some states, they can seek contraception or pregnancy care.

- In some states, they can seek outpatient mental health services.

- Abortion laws, as we know with the current state of politics, vary quite a bit from state to state with regards to the need for parental notification.

Let's talk further about the principle of autonomy (as it relates to minors), along with the principle of the child's best interest.

What if you had a 5-year-old patient and the parents declined polio vaccination? Let's contrast that particular situation with that of a 16-year-old who is in a car accident and requires a blood transfusion, but the parents refuse because their religion forbids a blood transfusion.

The approach is very different in these two cases. In the first case, parents are allowed to decline vaccination on behalf of their child. In the second case, the parents are not allowed to decline the blood transfusion because in this case it is a lifesaving intervention.

The main principle to remember is that of the child's best interest. In other words, is the proposed treatment in the child's best interest?

The reason why parents in the United States can refuse vaccination is that there's an acknowledgment that parents have the right to choose or refuse care for their children. Ultimately, parents are allowed to decide what happens to their children. An important point here: parents can only make these choices if they are considered competent in the eyes of the law. An abusive parent or a neglectful parent may have their decision-making rights terminated by the court.

The bottom line: If the parent is competent, they're allowed to make decisions on medical care, and that includes refusing medical care for their child. However, doctors can overrule these decisions if the medical intervention would either save the child's life or greatly enhance the quality of their life. That's why parents can refuse vaccination, but they can't refuse a lifesaving blood transfusion.

This may be straightforward in cases of life-saving treatment. But what about treatments that fall somewhere in the middle? Again, the principle to remember is that of the child's best interest. Will this treatment improve the child's quality of life? Is it likely to be successful?

For an interview question in which the treatment is one that falls in an "in-between" zone, the best path forward would be to discuss the situation with the parents and explain all the potential outcomes, both with and without the treatment. If the parents and the medical team disagree, then consultation with the hospital's Ethics Committee would be recommended. In some highly publicized cases, no agreement has been reached even after the Ethics Committee has weighed in. In some of those cases, the health care team had to bring the case to court.

Case #6

You are an oncologist who is asked to consult on a patient with recently diagnosed pancreatic cancer. He is a 75-year-old man with a history of severe depression. Although response to treatment is not guaranteed, there is a chance that chemotherapy may be beneficial. As you explain potential treatment options, he tells you that he is not interested in any treatment at all. What would you do?

Sample Answer

This is a very challenging case. On the one hand, physicians are committed to doing what is best for their patients, and it appears that chemotherapy may be helpful for this patient. However, the principle of patient autonomy is very important. Patients should be able to decide what type of medical treatment they will undergo.

I think this case is especially challenging because you mention that the patient has severe depression. The principle of autonomy applies to adult patients who have capacity, meaning they understand the different treatment options, the risks of those treatments, and the risks of not undergoing those treatments.

Therefore, I would first ask the patient more questions. Does he understand what will happen if he does not undergo any treatment? I would also ask if he would like include any family members or loved ones in our discussion. Next, I would ask for a psychiatry consult to understand what role his severe depression might be playing in his decision-making.

While I would respect the decision-making of a patient with the capacity to understand and make decisions about their medical care, I would make sure I had first gone through all of these steps.

Analysis

The student clearly lays out the main ethical concerns in this case.

Severe depression may interfere with the patient's capacity to understand the risks and benefits of treatment options.

The student clearly lays out the progression of what he would do in this case.

This concluding sentence emphasizes the need to understand a patient's capacity to make medical decisions.

Case #6: Key Points

Patient autonomy is one of the four major ethical principles that underlie medical ethics. Essentially, patient autonomy boils down to the concept that for an adult with capacity, it is their life and their body, and they get to decide what happens to it. Many times, this is a straightforward principle, but there are specific situations that are important to be aware of.

The principle of autonomy applies to an adult with capacity.

Complex Autonomy Scenarios

- What if your patient is a 16-year-old (not an adult) who is asking for an HIV test but does not want their parents to know that?
- What if you have a patient with Alzheimer's disease, and you're not sure if they can make this medical decision?
- What if it's an elderly victim of physical abuse who begs you not to call the police?
- What if it's a 45-year-old woman who's a victim of domestic abuse, who begs you not to call the police?
- What if it's a 39-year-old with a seizure disorder, who begs you not to report his seizure disorder to the authorities because then he won't be able to drive?

To answer these questions further, we have to delve a little bit deeper into the nuances of patient autonomy, so let's go back to our original case. This is a 75-year-old patient with severe depression who has been diagnosed with pancreatic cancer and who is now declining chemotherapy.

You need to be able to understand whether the patient has the capacity to make his decisions about his care. This question arises because the patient has severe depression and you're not sure if that is interfering with his capacity to make medical decisions. In this case, a psychiatry consult would be helpful.

Let's delve further into the concept of capacity because it's a key underpinning of autonomy.

Patients have capacity if...

- They can make a choice about their treatment and can communicate that choice.
- To do so, they need to be able to understand the diagnosis, prognosis, and the risk-benefit ratio of any of the proposed treatments, as well as the alternatives to those treatments.
- It's also important that any decision they make should be in harmony with what you know about their values.

How do you determine a patient's capacity to make these medical decisions?

First, it's very similar to the principle of innocent until proven guilty. A patient is presumed to have capacity unless a doctor can demonstrate otherwise. That's a very important concept. Questions arise when you're just not sure if a patient has that capacity to understand medical decisions. When that arises, often you can ask open-ended questions to see how much the patient understands.

For example, in the case of the patient with pancreatic cancer, you might say, "why do you think chemotherapy is not the right choice for you?" That will give you a little bit more insight into the patient's ability to understand the treatment, implications of the treatment, and alternatives to the treatments.

Ways to Determine Capacity

- Certain tests can help to assess capacity, and these include certain validated tools.
- There is not a minimum score on any test that can make this determination, so there are certainly gray areas when it comes to determining capacity.
- In some states two doctors must agree that a patient lacks capacity before you take away a patient's right to make their own medical decisions.
- That's a high bar—but it should be a high bar, because determining a patient's capacity is an important standard.
- Some patients clearly have capacity and other patients clearly do not. For example, a patient who has advanced dementia or psychosis clearly lacks medical decision-making capacity. In these patients, you would not need a psychiatry consult.

What are some of the reasons that a patient might not have the capacity to make their own medical decisions?

- Cognitive impairments such as advanced dementia can be one reason.
- Severe mental illness such as depression can be another one.

If a patient lacks capacity...

- A substitute decision-maker will be appointed.
- In some cases, a patient has already identified one via an advance directive such as a durable healthcare power of attorney.
- If they don't have an advance directive, then another substitute decision-maker will be identified.

Another important point to make about capacity is that it is decision-specific. For example, if somebody has Alzheimer's disease and they have fluctuating mental capacity, then you need to assess capacity every time you have to make a treatment decision.

You might also hear the term competency, but that is different than capacity. Competency is determined by a judge and it is a legal status. By contrast, capacity is determined by either one or two doctors' assessments and it doesn't carry a legal status.

Case #7

(Note: This case is included as a teaching case, not as a typical MMI scenario.)

You are working in the ER when you are asked to see your next patient. She is an 85-year-old woman who presents with a broken arm and multiple hematomas across her body. On deeper questioning, she explains that her son was angry with her and inflicted these wounds, but she does not want you to tell anyone. What would you do?

Would you inform the authorities? Or would you honor her wishes? Would you treat her injuries, but then encourage her to report her son to the authorities? Would you consult the Ethics Committee?

Sample Answer

In this case, an elderly woman is describing physical abuse by her son. This is a very upsetting and challenging case, because on the one hand you want to honor the patient's wishes, but on the other hand you have ethical and legal obligations.

Although patient confidentiality is important, legally and ethically, the physician is obligated to report elder abuse to the authorities. There are several situations in which physicians should breach patient confidentiality. Protecting vulnerable populations, such as children and the elderly, is one of those times.

I would therefore treat the patient's wounds. I would ask if there was another family member or loved one that could be with her as I was treating her. I would also contact the social work department and ask for additional support. Then, during treatment, I would gently explain to my patient that ethically and legally I am obligated to report the abuse to the authorities. I would reassure her that we had additional resources to help her, and I would be as supportive as possible.

Analysis

The student clearly outlines the ethical considerations here. "On the one hand... But on the other hand... "

Physicians need to be aware of the cases in which they should breach patient confidentiality.

Although we have a legal obligation here, it is important to focus on the care of the patient, and to provide compassion and support during this process. It is also important to connect the patient to additional resources.

Case #7: Key Points

This case centers on a particular aspect of autonomy, and that is the issue of a patient's privacy and right to confidentiality.

In general, a patient gets to decide when and with whom you (as the healthcare provider) share their medical information. However, there are times when ethically and legally you are required to breach patient confidentiality.

When to Breach Patient Confidentiality

1. For the public good
2. Child abuse
3. Elder abuse

The first reason you would breach confidentiality would be if it was in the "public good." For example, if you were treating a patient with a transmissible disease such as tuberculosis or a sexually transmitted disease such as syphilis, you would be required to report these to the health department. You are also required to report a patient who is expressing homicidal intentions.

There are other situations in which you're required to breach confidentiality, and these center on protection of the patient.

An important area for physicians is that of suspected child abuse. In cases of suspected child abuse, a physician is what is known as a "mandated reporter." As a physician, you are required to report your suspicions of child abuse, even if you don't have proof. If you have a suspicion, you need to report it. Other professions who work with children are also required to report suspected child abuse.

The elderly are also considered a vulnerable population, and therefore you are legally required to report cases of elder abuse.

Case #8

A 45-year-old woman presents with an arm fracture and multiple hematomas across her body. She reports that her husband had attacked her and caused these injuries, but she begs you not to tell anybody.

What do you do? Do you inform the authorities, or do you honor her wishes? Do you focus on treating her injuries and then encourage her to report her spouse?

Sample Answer

When I worked in the emergency room, we treated a patient who was a victim of domestic abuse. I learned a lot by watching the ER physician treat the patient, and we discussed the case afterwards.

I learned that in cases of domestic abuse, it is important to follow the patient's wishes and to respect their autonomy. Although other types of abuse must legally be reported to the authorities, such as child abuse and elder abuse, I learned that domestic abuse is considered a different category. That's because women in domestic abuse situations are not considered a vulnerable population.

In this case, therefore, the patient's right to autonomy would take precedence. I would focus on treating her injuries and then gently discuss her options further. Is there a family member or loved one that I could call to support her? Would she like to speak to a social worker? I would also provide her with information on more resources, including the number of a hotline and a shelter.

Although this is a challenging case, I would respect her autonomy but continue to provide support and information while encouraging her to report the abuse.

Analysis

The student describes her own experience with a similar case.

She clearly lays out the ethical and legal underpinnings of this case. One important point here: women in domestic abuse situations are not considered a vulnerable population, and therefore you do not have an obligation to override patient autonomy.

Although the patient has a right to autonomy, there are still multiple ways to support the patient and connect the patient to additional resources.

This concluding sentence summarizes the approach well.

Case #9

You are a family practice physician, and you have diagnosed a patient with a new-onset seizure disorder. The patient begs you not to report him to the authorities because if you do so, they will take away his car keys. In terms of mandated reporting, state laws vary.

Discuss the ethical issues involved here.

Sample Answer

I really feel for this patient, because apart from a very serious medical condition, he also has to contend with the potential loss of a valuable right. I think that most of us take the right to drive for granted, but I think of what it would be like to lose that right and to have to rely on others or on public transportation or on expensive ride-sharing services. Sometimes losing that right can even impact a person's ability to get to work and keep a job. That's a major consideration: how do reporting laws impact a person's quality of life and their ability to work?

In terms of medical ethics, on the one hand there is the issue of patient privacy. Patients are entitled to privacy of their medical information. However, there are times when physicians are required to breach patient confidentiality, so we also have to consider the public good. In this case, a major ethical concern is protecting the public from the risk of an impaired driver.

State laws likely vary because this is such a complex issue that encompasses these important issues of protecting the patient's quality of life and protecting their privacy versus protecting the public from the risks of an impaired driver.

Analysis

This opening statement empathizes with the patient's potential loss of a valuable right.

The major medical issues here center on patient privacy versus the public good.

Case #9: Key Points

In the United States there's not a clear-cut mandate to report a patient with a seizure disorder, and the laws vary by state.

In a clinical setting, the physician would focus on treatment for the seizure disorder and would encourage the patient not to drive. Depending on state laws, you would act appropriately.

This case goes back to the concept of patient confidentiality versus the public good. In certain cases, physicians are expected to break patient confidentiality because it is in the "public good," such as with certain transmissible diseases or if a patient expresses homicidal intentions.

Chapter 18:

Behavioral Interview Questions

Case #1

Tell me about a time you when you made a mistake and how you handled it.

Sample Answer

I was a new volunteer at the hospital, and they had a practice where we would give warm, scented towels to cancer patients to help with circulation and to let them freshen up and clear up their sinuses.

Being a new volunteer, I wanted to appear competent and show them that I was a great fit. On that first day that I was administering what is called oshibori—the warm scented towel—I made the mistake of giving a towel to a patient who had a sign on the door that said "no scents."

I realized the mistake the second I left the room. I closed the door and I saw the sign. I thought. "Oh my gosh, I messed up."

I reflexively felt that I needed to tell somebody about it. I needed to communicate it and let them know what happened; it was an honest mistake.

I did that. Thankfully, the nurse was very understanding, and thankfully for the patient, there was no harm done.

But what that did for me was to teach me that when I round, there are so many indicators for approaching a patient. I became more meticulous about how I round on patients. It also made me aware that it's okay to tell people about mistakes so we can get better and make sure it doesn't happen again.

Case #1: Key Points

This is an example of a behavioral interview question. They've been used for a long time in the business world, and they are increasingly used in medical interviews.

Proponents believe past behavior is a solid predictor of future behavior.

In answering questions like this, it's important to think about what is being asked. Though the interviewer has asked "tell me about a time when you made a mistake," the question should be "tell me about a time when you made a mistake…And how you handled it…And what you learned from it."

In answering this question, it's important to include all three components of this in your response.

Remember, this question is not about the mistake as much as it is about the interviewer wanting to learn how you deal with mistakes.

To answer behavioral interview questions, we recommend using the STAR approach.

The STAR Approach

- Situation: Describe the situation
- Task: In this example, the task is defined as, "how you are going to handle this mistake?"
- Action: What actions did you take to deal with your mistake?
- Results: What happened after you took action to deal with your mistake?

With the STAR approach, in essence, you are describing the situation and telling a story. It's helpful to include some details and background, without being too verbose.

As you think about what types of mistakes that you might discuss, it's best to avoid mistakes that have resulted in very bad outcomes because those mistakes can overshadow your lessons learned. You also want to avoid any stories that highlight character flaws.

The ideal mistake to discuss is one in which you demonstrated maturity in how you handled the mistake.

After you describe the results, it's very helpful to discuss lessons learned, and how you are planning to apply these lessons in the future. In the response here, note that the applicant has described a real mistake and how it impacted him. He concludes by describing the lessons learned. He uses words such as "what that did for me..." and "became much more meticulous."

Case #2

Tell me about a time when you had to deal with criticism.

Sample Answer

I was surprised by some criticism I received last year when I was shadowing an oncologist. The oncology team was very busy, and sometimes rounds stretched for over three hours. By the end of that stretch, my feet would be hurting, and sometimes I would lean against the wall to take some pressure off my feet.

One week into my experience, one of the oncologist's assistants took me aside. She was polite, but she made it clear that if I was not interested in this experience, then it would be best if I did not continue. I was surprised, because I was so grateful to have this incredible experience, and I was learning so much. I asked her why she felt that I was not interested, because that surprised me. She responded that the oncologist had noted that I often looked disinterested because he had noticed me slouched up against the wall.

I told her how surprised I was to hear this, and I told her that I had not realized that it would be perceived that way. I explained that I was leaning against the wall because of my tired feet. I told her that I could understand why it would be perceived as disinterest, but it definitely was not. She looked at me and said, "Oh, now that makes sense." She then said that she would go back to the oncologist and explain what had happened.

I also took it upon myself to write a thank you note to the oncologist, and I included a line about how grateful I was for the experience of shadowing and how interested I was in the cases that we were learning about. It had also come to my attention that my leaning against the wall because of my tired feet was giving the appearance that I was not interested, and that could not be further from the truth. I ended with a joke about how I was working on my podiatric endurance.

The assistant took me aside the next week and said that thanks to her explanation and my note, the physician now understood what had happened and was no longer concerned that I wasn't interested in rounds.

I was really thankful that the assistant had taken the time to approach me directly with her observations and perception. This is something that I think will be important throughout my career, especially in patient care. As a physician, I want to make sure that my patients always accurately perceive me as interested and actively listening. This really made me aware of the importance of nonverbal communication, and the importance of paying attention to my body language so that it is sending an accurate message. This is the lesson I'm going to keep with me throughout my career.

Case #2: Key Points

Since this is a behavioral interview question, you can utilize the STAR approach. After describing the situation, you want to identify the task. In this case, the task is, "how would you handle this criticism?"

You'll notice that in this response, the student has clearly outlined the actions he took to handle the criticism, from speaking to the assistant to writing to the physician.

With any behavioral interview question, it's also very helpful to clearly state the lessons learned. In this case, the student is making it clear that going forward, he will pay much greater attention to his nonverbal communication skills.

Case #3

Tell me about a time when you had to handle an uncomfortable situation with a colleague or coworker.

Sample Answer

Last summer, I began working as a waitress at a local restaurant. I was so excited to start working there, because it's an upscale restaurant known for its fantastic food. When I started this new position, I went through a training process that involved seven days of working with experienced waitstaff who would oversee my work for that day. On the fourth day, I was assigned to a waitress who was quite experienced. She had worked at the restaurant for over three years.

I arrived for my training shift, but as soon as I began working with her, I felt very uncomfortable. While the other waitstaff who had trained me had worked really hard to point out areas for improvement in a constructive way, this particular waitress almost seemed to revel in making me feel very small. Every time I made even a small mistake, such as placing the cutlery on the table in the wrong direction, she loudly corrected me. Although she never corrected me in front of the customers, as soon as we were out of earshot, she would turn to me and really let me have it.

I felt my stress level just rising and rising, and I just wasn't sure how to respond. I decided to just keep working to finish the tasks exactly the way she was directing me to. Essentially, I kept my head down and kept working hard while I was thinking about my next steps.

I knew that the manager might assign me to train under her for another shift, and I wasn't sure if I could handle it. I kept running different options in my mind, like speaking up right there or speaking to my manager.

However, I wanted to make sure that I completed my shift first. We finally finished our work at around midnight, so I decided to go home and really think about what I was going to say.

Two days later, when I returned for my shift, I asked her if she had a minute. I thanked her for helping to train me, and for paying such close attention to detail. I also commented on how much her customers seemed to love her, and how I admired that. However, I was wondering if there was anything I had done to upset or anger her, because some of her comments to me had seemed to indicate that.

Interestingly, she was surprised. She didn't realize that I felt that way, and I, in turn, was surprised that she didn't recognize her own behavior as harsh. She told me that she hadn't meant to be overly critical, but she found it very stressful to take care of her customers while she was training new waitstaff, and that's probably what I had sensed.

After that, things became easier. We ended up working the rest of the summer side-by-side, and although we never became close friends, after that she was always cordial to me.

This experience was uncomfortable, but I'm actually glad that I went through it, because it gave me a new perspective on uncomfortable situations. First of all, I did do something right: I was really glad that I had waited until after the shift was over and my emotions weren't running quite as hot when I approached her. I was also glad that I never lost my temper in front of the customers or during a busy shift, even when she was yelling at me.

One important lesson for me was that I learned what it's like to be on the receiving end of someone else's stressful day. I know that I never want to act like that to my own trainees or, later as a physician, to my staff or patients.

Chapter 19:

Traditional Interview Questions

One type of MMI station is the traditional interview question station. Although you might think of the MMI as focused on discussion questions or ethical questions, some stations are in fact devoted to traditional interview questions.

This question will be posted on the door, and when you enter, you'll sit down with the interviewer and answer the traditional interview question the same way you would during a traditional interview. For these stations, expect to give a shorter response, leaving much more time for follow-up questions and discussion with your interviewer.

Our companion book, the *Medical School Interview: Winning Strategies from Admissions Faculty* provides in-depth guidance to help you respond to traditional interview questions.

We've included an excerpt from the book that focuses on the very common traditional interview question of "Why did you apply to our medical school?"

Case #1

Why did you choose to apply to our medical school?
What qualities are you looking for in a school?
Describe your ideal medical school.
What interests you most about our school?
Tell me what you know about our school.
Why do you want to be a student here?
What two or three things are important to you in a medical school?

Typical Responses

"Well, I've lived here for three years so I know that I would want to live here. One of the things I like is the diversity and clinical opportunities you offer. I know I would see all kinds of different patient populations. The school has a good reputation which I know would help me get into a good residency program. The atmosphere is excellent, students help each other, and this is a place which will challenge me but not bring out the worst in me."

"I'm really looking for two things. First, a program that really integrates the clinical with the basic sciences. My impression is that [your school] does a good job with that. The second thing is the breadth of opportunities here. All the research that's going on. I can't imagine that it would be difficult to find many people I would be interested in working with."

"It seems like the school will help you reach your goals. You also have a lot of hospitals you can work at. Also, I'm interested in the International Health Track."

"I'll get a great education here. There are so many research opportunities. And students really seem to love the school. Also, the faculty is very involved with the students. Also having all the affiliated hospitals that you have here."

"The shorter basic science period really appeals to me. So does the way the basic science is structured, for example the way anatomy is spread over a number of semesters. I really like the medical center and Houston. The center is top notch."

What do all of these responses have in common?

They're all underwhelming. While there a number of reasons for this, the main one is that all of these applicants end up sounding pretty generic. The responses are fine and nobody's sending up any red flags, but at the same time you'd be hard pressed to remember any of these applicants.

Why is that?

First, most of these responses are too brief. Second, most of these responses lack specific details about the school, and all of them lack specific details about the applicant. Third, there's very little here that would convince the interviewer that this specific applicant would be a perfect fit with the school. And finally, there's nothing memorable in any of these responses. In other words, just about any applicant could have given the same response.

The biggest fail here is that every single applicant lost out on a valuable opportunity to impress the interviewer.

To see how a student could answer this question in a more compelling manner, let's meet Elena, an undergraduate student in Arkansas.

Elena's Story

Elena grew up in a medically underserved area with a significant Latino population. There were relatively few primary care physicians in her community, and even fewer specialists. Several of Elena's relatives passed away of cancer, and Elena developed an early interest in oncology. After finishing medical school, Elena hopes to pursue residency training in internal medicine followed by fellowship training in oncology. She plans to return to her hometown to practice oncology, and would be one of only two oncologists serving a four-county area. In college, Elena worked with Dr. Garcia, a dermatology faculty member at a local medical school, to develop an instructional module to help primary care physicians differentiate benign from cancerous skin lesions. The main goal was to provide a resource for primary care physicians practicing in parts of the state lacking access to dermatologists. Elena was also involved in organizing and implementing skin cancer screenings in these underserved areas.

Elena's Answer

"I first heard about your school from my faculty mentor, Dr. Garcia. Your school has an excellent reputation, and she spoke very highly of the education you offer. You're also well known for quality of teaching and diversity of patients, which I value. I also would love to live in Dallas, and have family in the Fort Worth area."

Analyzing Elena's answer

Be as specific as possible to confirm that your selection of their school was based on some thought and effort. Too often, applicants give a general answer. If you could give the exact same answer at another school, then your answer isn't good enough. If you examine Elena's response, you'll see that her answer, for the most part, was short on specifics. A better response is shown below.

Begin by researching the school thoroughly. What makes this school unique? What aspects of the school or its curriculum do you find particularly compelling? This information allows you to tailor your responses. In simple terms, if the school highly values research, and you have an interest or experience in that area, then you need to discuss it.

If a faculty member recommended the program, then by all means say so, as Elena did. Schools like to know that they're well regarded. Speaking with someone who has firsthand knowledge of the school also demonstrates that you've taken the time and initiative to learn as much as you can about the school. It demonstrates the seriousness of your interest.

There are also certain responses that you need to avoid at all costs. Avoid answers that confirm a disconnect between what you're seeking and what the school offers. Never put down another school. Lastly, while the geographic location of the school may be a major factor in your interest, avoid offering location as the only or initial reason for applying to the school.

Improved Answer

"I first learned about your school through my faculty mentor. Dr. Garcia is a graduate of your school and she's always spoken highly of the training she received. I would love to be a medical student at your school for a number of reasons. In shadowing physicians, I've learned that it's important to go to a school that places an emphasis on clinical skills. Your school has a reputation for being a leader in clinical skills development. The early patient contact, frequent observation of skills followed by regular feedback, and simulation lab are particularly appealing to me. It's also important to me that I develop a strong foundation for the practice of high quality care with patient safety in mind. That's why I'm really excited about your unique patient safety curriculum. And finally, I know that your school has a track for the underserved, and I could really see myself thriving in this track. In college, some of my most rewarding experiences occurred when I was involved in organizing and implementing health fairs for rural communities. Receiving education in caring for an underserved population would be fantastic because I would like to make this an important part of my future career in medicine. I grew up in a medically underserved area, and would like to return to my hometown as an internist and oncologist. On a personal note, I do have family in the Forth Worth area, and training in Dallas would allow me to spend time with family."

Chapter 20:

Scenarios Related to COVID

Case #1:

Your hospital has had several cases involving minors asking to be vaccinated for COVID without parental consent. You are asked to put together a hospital committee tasked with creating a set of guidelines for its staff when approached by such patients.

Sample Answer:

This is a very difficult issue, and during a pandemic, I would want to make sure that our committee acts quickly for the sake of our patients and for the sake of our community.
I would want to make sure that our committee examines this issue from several different perspectives, including the hospital's perspective, the minor's perspective, and the community's perspective.

In the short term, how would our staff handle a minor patient walking in and requesting a vaccination without their parents' consent? It's important to look at this from several perspectives. First, from the standpoint of the hospital system, legal issues are important. What does state law say? I know that in general, minors don't get to make their own medical decisions. However, there are exceptions that vary state by state, and I know these exceptions sometimes cover vaccinations. Since this varies by state, I would make sure that our committee included legal counsel. I would also make sure that our committee had medical ethicists, who could tell us more about issues concerning minors and medical consent.

It's also important to look at this from the patient's perspective. Our hospital's mission is to help our patients. How can we help this minor patient? If we can't legally administer the vaccine, can our committee provide assistance in other ways? I would explore other methods to reach vaccine-hesitant parents. I would consider an educational campaign that might involve reaching out to local media sources, as well as providing robust information on our website. For our patients, we might develop a website or brochure that specifically addresses this

Analysis:

The applicant lays out the framework of her response.

It is important to learn about the legal ramifications of this issue.

If legally the hospital is not able to provide vaccines, how else is the hospital able to help these minor patients? The applicant lays out several potential solutions.

issue. We might be able to provide resources on "how to talk to your parents about vaccination" and "legal resources for minors seeking vaccination."

In thinking about long-term considerations, our committee should learn more about community organizations that provide resources for minors seeking vaccination without parental consent. We may even need to explore the possibility of reaching out to lawmakers about our patient care experiences. I would include these voices on our committee.

Long-term considerations are important as well.

The most important thing is to assemble a team of experts so that we can legally and ethically help our young patients.

Case #1: Key Points

There have been some recently publicized cases of minor patients who wish to be vaccinated against their parents' wishes. These cases bring up several important ethical and legal issues.

Before we delve into these, it's important that physicians do everything they can to help preserve family relationships. This can mean encouraging your adolescent patient to have that conversation with their parents (if they feel safe doing so), or even helping to facilitate a family meeting.

In general, the principle of autonomy states that a patient gets to decide what medical care is provided to them, and therefore is allowed to decline medical care as well. However, this principle specifically applies to adult patients with the capacity to understand and make decisions about their medical care.

For minors, parents generally are the authorities deciding what medical care to provide for their children, as well as which medical care to refuse—with some notable exceptions. The laws related to these exceptions typically vary by state.

Can minors get vaccinated without parental permission?

In most areas, minors who are married or legally emancipated may provide informed consent for their own medical care

In general, minors who are pregnant may provide informed consent for their own medical care

Most states require parental consent for most healthcare decisions, including vaccination

A few states allow minors to become vaccinated without parental permission or notification

A few states only allow this for HPV and hepatitis B vaccines (because these two specific vaccines are considered to fall under rules related to sexually transmitted disease prevention and treatment)

Court intervention may also allow a "mature minor" to have autonomy over their medical decisions. Mature minors are adolescents who are clinically evaluated and are deemed competent to consent or refuse treatment

There has been a push to expand the laws providing permission for minors to consent to vaccination. By age 14, their cognitive capacity begins to align with adult decision-making. Particularly in the case of vaccination, it has been argued that minors should be allowed to consent to these highly beneficial and low-risk treatments, especially when their choices will advance their own health and the public health.

Ramifications to Be Aware Of

In general, the right for a minor to give consent also means a right to privacy. In other words, if you were allowed to vaccinate a minor without parental permission, you need not notify the parent

In general, either parent may consent to vaccinate their child, even if the other parent is known to have objections

If providing vaccination to a minor, it's important to consider how that vaccination will be paid for

---

If a minor is allowed to be vaccinated without their parents' permission, do you as the physician still have to notify their parents? This is an important question, and again, state laws vary. However, the general rule of thumb is if the minor has the legal right to give informed consent, then they also have the right to confidentiality.

What happens in cases where parents disagree on the medical care for their child? In most areas, either parent may consent to medical care even if the other parent objects. If parents are divorced or unmarried, it's important to look at custody agreements, because these sometimes contain specific procedures for medical care and consent.

Finally, it's very important to consider who will be paying for this vaccination. If paid for via health insurance, an explanation of benefits will be sent to the parents clearly outlining payment for the vaccination. Your patient needs to know about this before they proceed. If the minor patient does not wish to use health insurance, physicians can look for other resources to pay for the vaccines. There are programs that provide vaccines free of charge to children who cannot afford them.

References

Morgan L, Schwartz JL, Sisti DA. COVID-19 Vaccination of Minors Without Parental Consent: Respecting Emerging Autonomy and Advancing Public Health. *JAMA Pediatrics*. Published online July 12, 2021. doi:10.1001/jamapediatrics.2021.1855

Your Patient Bucks Parents on Vaccine Request. Now What? Accessed August 3, 2021. https://www.aafp.org/news/opinion/20190313guested-vaccines.html

Case #2

You are a medical student rotating on the internal medicine service in October 2020. This week, you are in the ICU. The clinical team is overseeing care of a patient positive for COVID. The attending physician asks the other medical student you are rotating with to check on the patient and take a brief history this morning. The other medical student refuses, telling the attending that she cannot catch COVID. The attending now turns to you and asks you to see the patient.

What are the ethical dilemmas presented in this scenario?

Sample Answer:

This scenario presents several ethical dilemmas, the first of which is the safety of healthcare professionals. To what extent are healthcare professionals expected to put themselves at risk to treat patients? Should healthcare professionals sacrifice themselves at any cost to patients? Just like patients, healthcare professionals are still people.

While they have taken an oath to do no harm, this does not mean they must save patients in all circumstances, such as in cases where it would result in extreme personal cost to the healthcare professional. For example, a respiratory ICU nurse who has an autoimmune condition, who is at great risk of dying if they are to contract COVID, has a legitimate personal concern.

At the same time, healthcare professionals still have a duty to care for their patients. What are the responsibilities of the healthcare system to protect its healthcare professionals? It is essential for the healthcare systems to protect healthcare providers in a pandemic as much as reasonably possible, such as providing personal protective equipment. However, it is also possible for personal protective equipment to be scarce in a pandemic—another ethical dilemma.

This scenario also begs the question, what are the responsibilities of a trainee? Trainees are a part of the medical community, and as such, they should be expected to contribute to care, even during a pandemic. Yet, just like attending physicians, trainees are also still people.

Analysis:

This response begins with the first ethical dilemma, focusing on the safety of healthcare professionals.

This delineates another ethical dilemma: what are the responsibilities of the healthcare system?

Another ethical dilemma relates to the responsibilities of trainees.

We do not know if the medical student who refused to see the patient in this scenario has a health condition which would increase her risk of getting very sick from COVID. This also brings in confidentiality, because we can't expect the medical student to reveal any medical conditions she has to the healthcare team. So, while the medical student has a right to refuse to see the COVID patient, assuming I am healthy and will be provided adequate personal protective equipment, I have a responsibility to see the patient when my attending asks me to.

With any scenario, we do have to consider other possible explanations. In this case, this may bring up the additional ethical dilemma of confidentiality.

In summary, this case addresses risks posed to healthcare workers, the responsibility of the healthcare system to protect its professionals, and the duty of healthcare trainees.

This conclusion summarizes the major ethical dilemmas of this case.

Case #2: Key Points

As a tenet of medical ethics, healthcare professionals have a right to legitimate personal interests. In other words, physicians need to balance their personal lives and health with their professional responsibilities. It is ethically acceptable for the physician to have concern for their own health and sacrifice some professional responsibility if it comes at a great personal cost.

Providers are expected to exercise their discretion when caring for COVID patients. They may be a member of populations who are at greater risk when caring for COVID patients, such as pregnant women or individuals with chronic medical conditions.

Pandemic ethics guide physicians to care for COVID patients, when personal protective equipment is available, as part of their professional duty. It is recommended to include trainees as a part of this professional responsibility.

Note the student brings in another ethical topic, confidentiality, to make the answer more comprehensive.

References

[1.] Giardino AP, Riesenberg LA, Varkey P. Medical Quality Management: Theory and Practice. Springer Nature; 2020.

[2.] Kramer JB, Brown DE, Kopar PK. Ethics in the Time of Coronavirus: Recommendations in the COVID-19 Pandemic. J Am Coll Surg. 2020;230(6):1114-1118. doi:10.1016/j.jamcollsurg.2020.04.004

Case #3

You are the nurse manager at a family practice clinic. Your patient, Mr. Markman, arrives for his appointment. He scheduled this appointment two days earlier for worsening swelling in his legs. He has a history of chronic obstructive pulmonary disease, along with hypertension and heart disease.

Because COVID cases in your community are rising, you have instituted a mask mandate in the clinic. The medical board of your state has also published a statement recommending that every medical facility in the state institute a mask mandate for all patients and healthcare providers.

As the receptionist was checking Mr. Markman in for his appointment, he told her that he refused to wear a mask. The receptionist explained that was the policy, but he still refused. She has now asked you to help.

Enter the room and speak with Mr. Markman.

Sample Answer

Nurse: Hello, Mr. Markman, I'm Elizabeth, the nurse manager here at the clinic. Jane, our receptionist, tells me that you do not wish to wear a mask. I want to make sure I understand the situation correctly. Can you tell me more?

Patient: I know that she said it was office policy, but I just really can't wear a mask. I have COPD, and I have a hard enough time breathing as it is. I can't make it worse by wearing a mask.

Nurse: That sounds really difficult, and I'm sorry to hear about your breathing difficulties. It is the clinic policy and the state policy for all medical facilities to have all patients and staff wear masks. Would you like to try one of our masks? We stock a particular brand that our patients have told us is soft and easier to handle.

Patient: I really don't want to try any mask at all. I've tried a lot of different ones, and they all cause the same problems. I just find it too hard to breathe.

Nurse: I understand, so let me work with you to try and find a solution. We have to be really careful, because we want to make sure that you are not exposed to the virus. As you know, it is present in airborne particles, which is why the mask is so important. At the same time, we also have to make sure our staff are protected as well. Would it be possible to reschedule you for a telemedicine appointment? We could make sure that you're seen by the physician later today.

Patient: I don't think that's going to work. I have a history of heart disease, and I have

Analysis

Although the manager has been told that "the patient refused to wear a mask", it's important not to jump to conclusions. The phrase "can you tell me more?" is a very helpful opening to this conversation.

The nurse expresses empathy. She also offers an alternative solution.

"Let me work with you to try and find a solution." There are medical reasons that interfere with a patient's ability to wear a mask, so it's important to work with the patient to provide medical care. Advances in telemedicine have been incredibly helpful during the pandemic.

worsening leg swelling, so I think the doctor really needs to examine my legs.

Nurse: It sounds like that would be necessary. Let me see if I can speak to the physician and try to work out a solution where you are in the office unmasked for as short a time as possible. I wonder if you could speak to the physician using your phone while sitting in your car, where you explain your medical history to the physician. Then, we could have you come into the office for a very short amount of time to do a targeted physical exam. After, we could send you back to your car and have the doctor speak to you by phone to explain what she found and come up with a treatment plan for you. If she thinks that that is a workable solution, would that work for you?

Patient: Yes, I think that would be okay, as long as the doctor is fine with it.

In this case, the nurse has come up with a hybrid model that will limit patient and physician exposure while still allowing for medical care.

Case #3: Key Points

As we read about in multiple news articles, enforcing mask mandates can be very challenging, especially for our frontline workers. Although such mandates may be required by healthcare facilities or by local or state agencies, it is understood that certain exceptions may need to be made.

In this case, it is important that the nurse manager began by trying to discover why the patient was refusing to wear a mask. It is important not to jump to conclusions. While there are many individuals who may refuse to wear a mask because of personal reasons or a fear that it is encroaching on their personal liberties, it is important to recognize that some patients may have medical reasons that interfere with their ability to wear a mask.

Once the nurse manager confirmed that the patient had an underlying pulmonary condition and was having difficulties breathing with the mask, her focus turned to finding a solution to the problem. In this case, the applicant demonstrated respect for the patient by calmly asking about their reasons for refusing to wear a mask. The applicant also demonstrated empathy and responded to the patient's comment that they were having difficulty breathing.

In cases like this, it's important to demonstrate to the patient that you are working to find a solution that will help the patient while still protecting the staff and vocalizing empathy as well.

Case #4

You are the leader of a large healthcare system. As vaccines developed to protect against complications of COVID have been shown to be safe and effective, your organization made the decision to institute a vaccine mandate. All employees will be required to receive the vaccine, with a few medical and religious exemptions.

How would you present this mandate to your workforce?

Sample Answer

Analysis

This is an important mandate, and it is truly a medical miracle that safe and effective vaccines have been developed and are now available for anyone in the United States.

However, we all know that there are many people in the United States who have declined vaccination, and my approach as the leader of my healthcare organization is to try to reach as many of those individuals as I can.

I would progress with a several stage approach.

This clearly describes the applicant's approach.

First, I would institute weekly emails to all of our employees. I would make these short and targeted. The first set would focus on incentives for vaccination, such as paid time off or free meal vouchers. Next, I would include photos of employees proudly showing off their vaccinations. I would also make sure to include statistics of how many of our employees were vaccinated, in order to make it clear that this is "normal" behavior for our employees. I would also advertise employee Town Halls, where we would answer any questions about vaccine development and safety.

The use of transition words such as "first" and "next" is helpful in structuring the response.

At the same time, I would start a public relations campaign talking about how our employees are health heroes. I saw this kind of poster when I visited the hospital last month, and it had a big superhero picture with a caption saying that their vaccinated employees were health heroes because they were protecting their patients. I would really double down on that message that we are healthcare professionals and health heroes, and we get vaccinated because we are

The applicant describes a tactic used by another hospital.

protecting our immunocompromised and vulnerable patients.

In the final stage, I would move onto information about our upcoming vaccine mandate. I would point out that our hospital system has always required vaccinations, such as hepatitis B vaccinations for all of our employees and the flu vaccine every year, and that the COVID vaccine will similarly also be required. I would make sure to tell any employees who were still hesitant that we had a special page on our website to answer any questions that they had. Finally, I would make it clear that our vaccine would be required by this date, and anyone who objected would be asked to leave the organization.

This is a strong argument supporting the legality of vaccine mandates for employees.

Ultimately, I would work with my team to outline our timeline for this progression, going from vaccine information, to incentives, to honoring our vaccinated employees as health heroes, to finally implementing our vaccine mandate.

In the conclusion, the applicant summarizes her proposed systematic approach to the vaccine mandate.

Promotion of COVID Vaccination Mandates for Healthcare Workers: Three Main Points

- First, we have a general ethical duty to protect others.
- Second, as healthcare workers we bear special ethical responsibilities that come from caring for patients.
- Third, there is a clearly established use of vaccine mandates for healthcare workers, such as for Hepatitis B and influenza.

Case #4: Key Points

All of us have a general ethical duty to protect others. This duty is even more imperative when the risk from vaccines to us is minimal, but the benefit to others is significant.

Second, anyone who works in the health professions, whether a front-line worker or behind the scenes, has a special ethical responsibility to protect the health and well-being of others.

Working in a healthcare setting means that these workers are more likely to interact with individuals who are vulnerable to COVID-19. For example, some of my patients receive certain immunosuppressive medications, and this may affect the protection offered by vaccines. One of my patients told me that she had her antibody titers tested after two doses of the Pfizer vaccine, and she did not produce antibodies. Studies have also shown that elderly adults may mount a less robust immune response. Finally, at the time of this writing, no vaccine has been approved for children under the age of 12 years.

The third main point is that requiring vaccination for healthcare workers is an established policy. Years ago, when I entered medical school, I was required to show proof of vaccination against hepatitis B as well as multiple other vaccines. This proof of vaccination has been a requirement for every job and at every hospital at which I have worked. The hospitals on which I serve as staff require flu vaccines every year for all of their staff members (with certain religious and medical exemptions).

Organizations that promote vaccine mandates have made it clear that vaccine mandates are legal. "As the US Equal Employment Opportunity

Commission has made clear, employers have the right to require vaccination as a condition of employment. This right extends to vaccines under emergency use authorization as well as those that have been fully approved by the FDA."

Organizations have also pointed out that mandates work. The Houston Methodist Hospital, where I am proud to serve on medical staff, was the first in the nation to require its employees to be vaccinated. It received backlash in the media, but in a message to all its employees, emphasized its commitment to "leading medicine." As the leadership explained, sometimes leading medicine can lead to uncomfortable situations, but it is important to do what is right for our patients. After the mandate, over 99% of employees received the vaccine, with only a small percentage resigning.

Vaccine hesitancy has been a major obstacle in the fight against COVID. In speaking to patients and employees, it is important to point out that this vaccine was not developed overnight. Just like many actors, the vaccine was not "an overnight success." Instead, basic science researchers have been performing the underlying scientific research for over a decade to support these vaccine platforms. That's the reason this vaccine appears to be an overnight success: it was over a decade in the making. Once the threat was clear, thousands and thousands of dedicated individuals came together to produce and make the vaccine accessible. Now, literally hundreds of millions of people have been safely vaccinated.

Importantly, this vaccine has dramatically reduced the risk of severe disease, hospitalization, and death. With that combination of vaccine safety and protection against a deadly disease, healthcare organizations are rightfully using every tool at their disposal to protect their employees as well as their patients.

References

Emanuel EJ, Skorton DJ. Mandating COVID-19 Vaccination for Health Care Workers. Annals of Internal Medicine. https://www.acpjournals.org/doi/10.7326/M21-3150. July 30, 2021.

U.S. Equal Employment Opportunity Commission. EEOC Issues Updated COVID-19 Technical Assistance. 28 May 2021. Accessed at www.eeoc.gov/newsroom/eeoc-issues-updated-COVID-19-technical-assistance.

Case #5

You are a family practice physician, and one of your longtime patients, Mrs. Smith, has scheduled a routine physical examination. She is 32 years old and healthy. When you ask her about her vaccination status for COVID, she states she is not interested in getting the vaccine. She has heard it causes infertility and is worried.

How do you discuss this issue with her?

Sample Answer

When I first read about patients refusing vaccination because of the risk of infertility, I was surprised. How could people believe these reports, when we have no evidence that the vaccine causes these types of side effects? Then, I found out that one of my cousins, who is in his 20s, had read about this same concern on social media and refused to get the vaccine. This changed my perception of the problem because it highlighted how even highly-educated individuals could believe in medical misinformation.

Overall, when it comes to medical misinformation, I have read that there are different ways to attack this problem. This might include national measures, community measures, and person-to-person measures.

In this case, since Mrs. Smith is one of my long-term patients, I believe there is a chance I could reach her. Reports have found that some vaccine-hesitant patients changed their minds after speaking to their physicians.

To address her vaccine hesitancy, I would start by listening and asking her more about her beliefs. I would explore where she gathered her information from and why she believed these supposed reports.

I would use active listening techniques, making sure that she felt heard and felt that I was taking her concerns seriously. I would use statements such as "I can see why you would be worried after reading that on social media." I would then explain the robust safety data that we have on the vaccines. "I can see why you might be concerned. However, let me reassure you about the safety data that we have."

Analysis

The applicant begins by sharing her own personal experience with vaccine hesitancy.

Despite prevalent social media misinformation, healthcare providers remain trusted sources for medical information.

Understanding the patient's beliefs can be very helpful in formulating a response and rebuttal.

While I would discuss some of the statistics behind the safety data, I would keep them simple and focused on individuals like her. For example, I might start by telling her about the tens of millions of people in the United States who are her age and have safely received the vaccine. If I learned where she obtained her information from, I would try to point out politicians or celebrities with whom she might identify that had been vaccinated.

Instead of a recitation of statistics, trying to make the data as personal to the patient as possible is a useful technique.

Additionally, I have read that telling people about former vaccine skeptics who changed their mind may in some cases be an effective technique. I would say something along the lines of: "It can be scary when you read about things like this on social media. There was a recent news report about one of our local community members who was also worried, but then changed their mind and is now urging others to get the vaccine. I can send you a link to the video if you like."

This is an additional technique that has been described in the literature on vaccine hesitancy.

Finally, I would tell her how worried I am about her health and safety, and this is why I am urging her to get vaccinated. I would tell her about how I had seen several of my long-term patients who had suffered from COVID, which is why I wanted to discuss vaccination with her. I would end by telling her that if she is not ready today, she can always contact the office and I can schedule her for vaccination. I would also tell her that if she had any future questions about the vaccine, she could reach out to me.

Many times, the conversation around vaccine safety can obscure the dangers of the disease. Bringing the focus back to the danger and tragedy of COVID by sharing the physician's own personal experiences with their patients can be an important technique.

Case #5: Key Points

How do you encourage a patient who is vaccine hesitant to proceed with vaccination?

In the midst of a global pandemic, this is an incredibly important and urgent question. There are no clear answers, and research is ongoing. This research is trying to determine underlying reasons for vaccine hesitancy, as well as potential interventions that can overcome that hesitancy.

One survey of unvaccinated patients describes a spectrum of vaccine hesitancy. Patients may be "vaccine ready", "vaccine neutral" or "vaccine resistant." The survey also further delineated those patients who were "vaccine ready" into those who were either actively seeking vaccination or those who were prepared to accept vaccination, as long as it involved minimal effort.

For some patients, then, providing easy access to vaccination may be critical. For patients who are vaccine neutral, a recommendation from their trusted physician may make all the difference. In one survey, for example, 15% of unvaccinated respondents said that they would be more inclined to be vaccinated if their healthcare provider recommended it to them.

In another study, the Kaiser Family Foundation surveyed a group of American adults who had originally said that they did not plan to get vaccinated, but then later decided to proceed with vaccination. In the survey, this group was known as "vaccine converts," and they were asked about what had made them change their minds.

Reasons for Proceeding with Vaccination: 3 Main Themes

1. Vaccine safety. Being able to see that millions of other Americans had been safely vaccinated helped sway them.
2. Hearing directly from people they knew who were sharing pro-vaccine messages. This included messages from doctors, friends, and family members.
3. The fear of being excluded from activities because they were not vaccinated. The urge to visit certain restaurants, events, or travel destinations that required vaccination helped sway some individuals.

What do the experts recommend? In an article by the American Medical Association on COVID vaccine hesitancy, experts shared their tips for speaking to patients. These recommendations included:

- Asking why a patient is declining the vaccine, and specifically asking "What have you heard in your community?" This is considered a less judgmental way to understand a patient's thoughts on the vaccine, because it gives them the chance to attribute any concerns they might have to others.

- Speaking to the patient as a physician and actively countering any misinformation. Some researchers have found that an individual's own physician or healthcare provider is often considered the most trusted source of information on the COVID vaccine.

- Going beyond just providing information and actually telling patients that they need to get the vaccine. In another study on barriers to adult immunization, adult patients said that the second biggest reason they didn't get an immunization was that a doctor "hadn't told me I needed it."

- Emphasizing the patient's ability to protect others, such as a child or someone who is immunocompromised. Concern for loved ones can often sway individuals when personal considerations haven't been as effective.

- Preparing patients for side effects of the vaccine, but emphasizing that these are similar to those of other vaccinations. Physicians can ask patients about what types of side effects they have experienced from other vaccinations, such as the flu vaccine. This provides a natural progression to then discuss the fact that the COVID vaccine is very similar in terms of side effects.

Another important point that experts emphasize is that moving a patient from vaccine hesitancy to vaccine acceptance may require a series of visits.

References

Leonhardt D. Vaccine Persuasion. *The New York Times*. https://www.nytimes.com/2021/07/19/briefing/vaccine-skepticism-vaccination-drive.html. Published July 19, 2021. Accessed August 4, 2021.

Ratzan S, Schneider EC, Hatch H, Cacchione J. Missing the Point — How Primary Care Can Overcome COVID-19 Vaccine "Hesitancy." *New England Journal of Medicine*. 2021;384(25):e100. doi:10.1056/NEJMp2106137

COVID-19 vaccine hesitancy: 10 tips for talking with patients. American Medical Association. Accessed August 4, 2021. https://www.ama-assn.org/delivering-care/public-health/COVID-19-vaccine-hesitancy-10-tips-talking-patients

Case #6

The United States has been criticized for its response to the COVID pandemic. Discuss measures taken by other nations around the world that provide important lessons for future pandemics.

Sample Answer

The COVID pandemic has led to so many tragic outcomes, and it's so unfortunate that we're still in the middle of so much suffering. I think there are important lessons to learn from how other countries around the world successfully implemented certain strategies to combat the pandemic.

I think one country to look to is New Zealand. Although the United States is, of course, not an island, one lesson from New Zealand is that they took the threat very seriously. From what I've read, they looked at models of the spread of COVID and realized that it would overwhelm their healthcare system. That led them to quickly institute a travel ban and a lockdown. Looking at reports from scientists and then acting quickly on those reports led them to have one of the most successful responses in the world.

I think we can also learn a lot from Taiwan. Although their citizens are more used to government surveillance, their emphasis on testing, contact tracing, and quarantining helped limit deaths from COVID. Especially with a virus that can be spread by asymptomatic individuals, the use of contact tracing is known to be very important. They also ramped up their production of personal protective equipment and have even been able to send medical supplies to other countries.

In terms of vaccination, Israel has been a model for the world. One of the reasons they were able to have quick access to vaccines is because they were willing to pay more, but it's now felt that that investment has been worth it. Their healthcare system is also more centralized than in the United States, which

Analysis

This is a well-structured response. The prompt asks for a discussion of measures taken by other nations that provide important lessons, and the applicant has started with one lesson from another nation.

She has moved on to another lesson: the importance of testing, contact tracing, and quarantining.

She is describing the importance of the logistics of a vaccination drive.

helped with their successful vaccination drive. Regardless, their focus on the logistics of quickly vaccinating a large part of their population carries important lessons.

Finally, I think that many countries across the world are struggling with the same medical misinformation on social media that the United States has had to contend with. Other countries, however, have seen their leaders focus on more consistent messaging. In the United States, the messaging from the leaders of the Navajo nation has been to protect the elders. Other leaders have strongly promoted masks, social distancing, and vaccines. With some of our politicians taking advantage of the strong polarization in this country, it has been challenging to stay on message.

As the United States continues to deal with the tragic consequences of this pandemic, many healthcare leaders are already thinking about how we can better respond to future crises. I think these lessons, of early action, extensive testing, vaccination, and especially strong messaging from leadership, will be very important.

This summary sentence clearly describes the lessons to focus on: early action, extensive testing, vaccination, and strong messaging.

Case #6: Key Points

There are a number of very important lessons to learn from other countries in terms of national responses to the COVID pandemic. These include responses related to:

- Early action
- Travel bans
- Widespread testing
- Contact tracing
- Quarantines
- Ramping up production of personal protective equipment
- Increasing capacity in the healthcare system (hospital beds, ICU beds, ventilators, ECMO) to provide care for patients with COVID
- Cultural messaging supporting the use of masks and social distancing
- Clear, decisive messaging from leadership on the importance of protecting others
- Clear, decisive messaging from leadership on the importance of masks, social distancing, and vaccination
- Combating medical misinformation on social media
- Vaccination

Some of these strategies and policies are more feasible for some nations than others. For example, nations with citizens who are more used to governmental surveillance may report greater adherence to contact tracing. Nations with citizens who are more used to governmental control may be able to institute dramatic and extremely strict quarantines, such as were seen in China. Island nations such as Singapore and New Zealand may be able to enforce travel bans more effectively.

Having said that, there are important lessons from both the policies and the results from multiple nations. These are incredibly important lessons that we are likely to have to implement again in the future.

Dr. Tom Frieden, former Director of the CDC (2009 to 2017), has written about what we can learn from the responses of nations worldwide to the COVID pandemic.

New Zealand has been held up for its strong and early response to the threat. It is an island, which of course makes it easier to enforce border controls. Regardless, their leadership acted quickly and decisively. When scientists modeled what community spread would look like, they determined that it would overwhelm their healthcare system. They also did not have the ability to test extensively and perform extensive contact tracing. Therefore, their leadership took early action to lock down the country and close their borders. (They also began preparing their hospitals.) These actions were felt to be the key to their earlier recovery from the pandemic and lower mortality than almost all other developed nations.

Taiwan also took early action. While they closed the borders to China, they also focused on widespread testing and increasing their production of personal protective equipment.

Similarly, South Korea acted quickly. One of the key lessons from their response was the importance of testing and extensive contact tracing. Especially with a virus such as COVID, where asymptomatic individuals can spread the virus, contact tracing becomes very valuable.

Of course, one of the most important facets of combating a pandemic is having clear messaging from leaders on the actions that its citizens should take. Some countries in Asia have a longer history of mask use, and so culturally this was adopted very quickly. Other leaders talked about the importance of masking in order to protect the elders of the community, such as in the Navajo nation. Finland has had strong initiatives to combat misinformation on social media. Unfortunately, in the United States public health messaging has been taken to have political implications. This has led to polarization on such basic topics as the importance of social distancing, the use of masks, and the benefits of vaccines.

Economic protection is also a strategy to contain pandemics. The United States expanded unemployment benefits and instituted a moratorium on evictions. These social services function as an important public health strategy, as they helped many individuals who otherwise would not have been able to adhere to lockdowns. Many nations across the world worked to protect their citizens. Denmark, for example, acted to avoid layoffs in the private sector by providing governmental support to cover employee salaries.

Vaccination is, of course, vital to ending the pandemic. Israel has been held up as a model of successful vaccination. Part of this success was due to leadership emphasizing the importance of vaccination and approving funding to have early access to these vaccines. Israel also has strong health management organizations that have centralized data-keeping and technology, which allowed the government to ramp up their vaccination drive quickly. They were able to target citizens with messages on vaccination via text, email, and phone. Although critics point out the implications of governmental access to medical information, this centralized technology did help with vaccination. Israel also improved vaccination via a tiered "passport" system, in which bars and restaurants were open to those who were vaccinated, providing an extra "nudge" to the unvaccinated.

References

As COVID-19 hits Navajo Nation, young people step up to protect elders. STAT. Published May 26, 2020. Accessed August 10, 2021. https://www.statnews.com/2020/05/26/navajo-nation-COVID-19-youth-response-elders-health/

Frieden T. Which Countries Have Responded Best to COVID-19? *Wall Street Journal*. https://www.wsj.com/articles/which-countries-have-responded-best-to-COVID-19-11609516800. Published January 1, 2021. Accessed August 10, 2021.

The Best Global Responses to COVID-19 Pandemic, 1 Year Later | Time. Accessed August 10, 2021. https://time.com/5851633/best-global-responses-COVID-19/

Policy Responses to COVID19. IMF. Accessed August 10, 2021. https://www.imf.org/en/Topics/imf-and-COVID19/Policy-Responses-to-COVID-19

Chapter 21

MMI And Your Future

As evidence supporting the multiple mini interview process in medical school admissions has accumulated, educators have started to examine the potential role of this interview format in residency admissions. Below we have listed and described some studies and their findings:

- In one study performed at a single family medicine residency program, the MMI was found to be a useful way to assess characteristics and behaviors valued in residents.[1]

- Researchers in Pennsylvania found the MMI process to yield reliable results among internal medicine residency applicants. Surveys of faculty and applicants showed that the format was preferred over the traditional interview.[2]

- Several programs in emergency medicine have adopted the MMI in their residency selection process. A recent article discussed whether the format addressed stakeholder needs.[3]

- At a Pediatric Academic Societies Meeting, Dr. Mona Attisha, Program Director of the Pediatric Residency Program at Hurley Medical Center, shared the findings of her research utilizing MMI in the residency selection process. She found that MMI data allowed for more informed rank-order decisions and was more predictive of future performance.[4]

- A study utilizing the MMI in the otolaryngology residency selection process found good reliability. Researchers also noted that the approach was considered acceptable to all major stakeholders.[5]

What does this mean for you? It may be that you will likely encounter the MMI again when it comes time to apply for residency.

References

[1]Hofmeister M, Lockyer J, Crutcher R. The acceptability of the multiple mini interview for resident selection. *Fam Med* 2008; 40 (10): 734-40.

[2]Fraga J, Oluwasanio A, Wasser T, Donato A, Alweis R. Reliability and acceptability of a five-station multiple mini-interview model for residency program recruitment. *Community Hosp Intern Med Perspect* 2013; 3 (3-4): 10.

[3]Phillips A, Garmel G. Does the multiple mini-interview address stakeholder needs? An applicant's perspective. *Ann Emerg Med* 2014; 64 (3): 316-9.

[4]Hanna-Attisha M, Cederna-Meko C, Campe B. Modified multiple mini interview (3MI): An effective & efficient approach for screening critical milestones during resident selection. Presented at Pediatric Academic Societies Poster Session (Publication 1533-510), Vancouver 2014.

[5]Campagna-Vaillancourt M, Manoukian J, Razack S, Nguyen L. Acceptability and reliability of multiple mini interviews for admission to otolaryngology residency. *Laryngoscope* 2014; 124 (1): 91-6.

For more on traditional medical school interview and behavioral interview questions, please see

MEDICAL SCHOOL INTERVIEWING 101

Quickly and confidently get the expert answers you need with our online course

With before-and-after videos and our step-by-step approach to help you craft personalized, unique responses to over 25 medical school interview questions

Our goal is to help you go from good to great to unforgettable

www.TheInterviewCourse.com

An excerpt from the best-selling book:
Success in Medical School:
Insider Advice for the Preclinical Years

By Dr. Samir P. Desai
and Dr. Rajani Katta

The Preclinical Years Of Medical School

Note: The following chapter is excerpted from the book – Success in Medical School: Insider Advice for the Preclinical Years

The preclinical years of medical school are extremely challenging, and that may be understating the reality. At one medical school, faculty assigned "29,239 pages of reading for the 12 basic science modules that bewere scheduled during 71 weeks."[1]

As you begin med school, you'll hear a lot of advice.

- "If you thought the MCAT was tough, wait until you see the USMLE."

- "The material it took you a semester to cover in college? You'll get through that in a week in med school."

- "If you want to go down the ROAD, you'd better start planning now, figure out your research, and make your connections early - and you'll have to maximize that first summer off." [ROAD = Radiology, Ophthalmology, Anesthesiology, Dermatology]

There is at least some truth in every one of those statements.

Medical school is extremely challenging, and not just in the ways that you'd assume. The sheer volume of material covered is staggering. And most importantly, unlike in some of your college courses, much of it builds upon prior material. Your study methods therefore have to ensure long-term retention. In Chapter 2 [Preclinical Courses], you'll hear advice from students, faculty, and experts, as well as the results of research, on how to learn such a large volume of material, and how to ensure retention. In one study, researchers found that "in general, study skills are stronger predictors of first-semester total grades than aptitude as measured by the MCAT and undergraduate GPA."[2] The importance of long-term retention of basic science material is emphasized by the United States Medical Licensing Exam. The USMLE Step 1 exam is taken at the end of the preclinical years, and your score on this single exam can influence the course of your career. The exam tests your ability to take the basic science material covered over two years in medical school and apply it to clinical situations. In Chapter 3, you'll learn about the exam itself, as well as the most common mistakes that students make when preparing. You'll learn about resources that can aid your preparation, and you'll learn about the importance of this single score in the residency application process. Chapter 4 provides specifics about the COMLEX Level 1 exam. This exam, taken by osteopathic students, is of similar importance.

While mastering such a large amount of basic science material is extremely challenging, unfortunately that's not enough. Your skills in the hands-on art and science of patient care will be critical. Learning about a disease and its manifestations in the classroom does not ensure that you'll know what to do when faced with a patient in the clinic. It is widely believed that physicians' examination skills have deteriorated over the years. While a number of factors may be responsible, it is believed that clinical skills training may play a role. In fact, if you don't adequately learn certain skills and techniques during your preclinical courses [Introduction to Clinical Medicine or Physical Diagnosis], you may never learn them, not even during clerkships. "Surveys have indicated that less than 16% of attending time may be spent at the patient's side."[3] This has important ramifications for patient care. When researchers observed interns and residents, they noted frequent errors in physical exam technique, including improper use of instruments. In Chapters 5 [Taking a Patient History] and 6 [Physical Examination], you'll learn how to make the most of your history and physical exam education.

The challenges of the preclinical years extend beyond the well-known. Chapters 11 and 12 provide some startling statistics on medical student well-being and issues of professionalism. Physicians are challenged on a daily basis with the stressors of clinical patient care, and the coping mechanisms and buffering strategies you develop now, as a preclinical student, will be vital throughout the course of your career.

Several chapters highlight the significant opportunities available to medical students. Medical schools, organizations, and individual medical students have all been able to impact medical practice or their communities in significant ways, and their accomplishments are inspiring. Chapters on Community Service, Extracurricular Activities, and Research serve as a guide on how to get started, and highlight the numerous opportunities for preclinical students to become involved and thus have the opportunity to make a meaningful impact. Chapters on teaching, awards, and international experiences provide details on further opportunities.

Throughout these challenges, you do have to consider your future. As the residency selection process for certain fields becomes ever more competitive, students who have at least started strategizing early in their education will be at an advantage. Chapter 16 [Choosing a Specialty] reviews the process of strategizing in detail. For the most competitive specialties, great grades and high USMLE scores are not enough. You'll need great letters of recommendation and support from faculty advocates. In Chapter 10 [Mentoring], you'll learn ways in which preclinical students can approach established faculty members and obtain their assistance and guidance. You'll also need additional distinctions. Most applicants to the competitive specialties will have performed research, and many will have publications or presentations to their name. Chapter 7 [Research] reviews the process, demonstrates how students can begin, details what to seek in a research project, and provides specifics on research, publication, and presentation opportunities available to medical students. Some residency programs also seek additional factors of distinction, such as involvement in extracurricular activities, evidence of leadership, and commitment to service. In "Choosing a Specialty," you'll learn how to start the process of exploring a specialty. The chapter also includes specifics about identifying research opportunities, locating specialty-specific mentors, seeking out community service projects within the field, and other specialty-specific opportunities.

Throughout the next 300+ pages, we'll review each of these areas in detail. From grades and exams, to the art of patient care, to strategizing for your career, you'll learn specific, detailed information relevant to the preclinical medical student. These reviews and recommendations are based on the experiences of students, residents, and faculty, as well as a thorough review of the scientific literature in the areas of medical education and patient care. This combination of insider information and evidence-based advice is utilized to help you gain the strongest foundation as you face the challenges of medical school. Your goal is to become the best doctor possible, and that process begins on day one of medical school.

Preclinical courses/grades

At one medical school, faculty assigned "29,239 pages of reading."[1]

The core of this chapter centers on one vital question related to that startling fact. How can a student read and retain such a large volume of information?

In Chapter 2, you'll learn what students, faculty, and experts advise on how to get through the mountain of material a med student is expected to master. The most common mistake that med students seem to make? They assume that studying longer and harder will be enough to succeed.

It's not.

The students who are able to excel in medical school have learned how to effectively strategize and utilize the techniques of active learning, among other study strategies. Reading and highlighting material, even multiple times, won't be enough to ensure the long-term retention that medical school requires.

Upperclassmen at the University of Alabama Birmingham School of Medicine offer the following advice to new students: "The material is rarely difficult; there is just a mountain's worth to cover. A normal medical school exam seems like a cumulative final in the most strenuous science course you took in undergraduate. You simply cannot learn the material overnight or with one quick read-through of the scripts."[4]

Prior to med school, you no doubt heard about the heavy academic workload. The volume of material to be covered is truly enormous, and while students expect this, it doesn't fully sink in until the first week when you receive lecture materials, syllabi, and books. Consider the following comments made by new medical students:

- "I was worried that I wouldn't be able to keep up."

- "What scared me most was the amount of information I was asked to master."

- "It was all so overwhelming. How could I possibly learn it all? After all, I could barely carry it."

While the preclinical curriculum will vary among medical schools, most schools will focus on the same core subjects. In 2006, the International Association of Medical Science Educators convened a group of respected medical educators to answer some key questions about the role and value of the basic sciences in medical education.[5] The educators identified eight sciences - anatomy, physiology, biochemistry, neuroscience, microbiology, immunology, pathology, and pharmacology – as "vital foundations of medical practice." Also deemed critical to a strong foundation was education in behavioral sciences, genetics, epidemiology, molecular biology, and biostatistics.

Given the significant challenges of learning and retaining this much material, what is the best way for students to approach their preclinical courses? In this chapter, you'll learn the differences between top and average performers, and you'll learn about study strategies that have led to success. In one study, researchers found that "in general, study skills are stronger predictors of first-semester total grades than aptitude as measured by the MCAT and undergraduate GPA."[2] You'll learn about common mistakes that students make when approaching the basic sciences, and how to avoid those mistakes. You'll also hear suggestions from students who have successfully navigated these challenges.

Taking a Patient History

It's well-known that the transition between learning about medicine in the classroom and actually applying that knowledge in the care of real patients is quite challenging. Studies have confirmed that students have high levels of stress and anxiety as they move from the preclinical to clinical years of medical school.[14]

Clinical skills, including the history and physical exam, are often mentioned as a major struggle in the transition period. One student described her discomfort. "I felt uncomfortable talking to the patient and trying to come up with methodical ways of asking questions and making sure I didn't miss things, not just jumping around all over the place."[15]

Traditionally, preclinical students have had limited contact with patients. In recent years, however, schools have placed new emphasis on clinical skills training in early medical education. Some schools now even introduce students to patients as soon as the first week or month of medical school.

Medical organizations have also recognized the importance of an early emphasis on clinical skills, including communication. In 2004, the Institute of Medicine made the acquisition and development of communication skills a top priority during medical education. That same year, the National Board of Medical Examiners (NBME) began requiring students to take a clinical skills exam (USMLE Step 2 CS) as a means to assess competence in communication. The hope is that through education on effective communication, students will be better versed in how to listen, question, counsel, and motivate patients.

Your efforts to improve communication skills will also impact your clerkship performance. In a survey of clerkship directors, while over 95% felt that students require an intermediate to advanced level of communication skills, approximately 30% felt that new clerkship students aren't sufficiently prepared.[16]

Medical schools evaluate communication skills in different ways. One is through comprehensive clinical skills assessment using standardized patients. Researchers have interviewed faculty members responsible for helping those students who don't perform well in these assessments. Some of the issues have focused on patient histories.[17] "Many low-scoring students focused prematurely, failing to ask open-ended questions or adequately characterize the chief complaint. Respondents also observed students being too focused on the history of present illness, omitting or incompletely exploring the pertinent past medical, social, or family history, particularly as they related to the chief complaint." Some students failed to explore the patient's perspective on the illness. The authors wrote that "these students treated standardized patients as symptoms or diagnoses rather than as people with feelings or concerns."

In Chapter 5, you'll learn how to make the most of your clinical skills education. You'll learn about the deficiencies that have been documented in the physician-patient communication literature with respect to history taking, and how educators have developed benchmarks to guide medical students in their acquisition of important communication skills. As you develop your history taking skills, you'll learn how to use these benchmarks, solicit feedback to assess your progress, and reflect on your own performance in order to improve your skills.

Physical Examination

Although 80% of diagnoses are made based on the history and physical examination, evidence indicates that the physical exam skills of physicians today are inadequate. It is widely believed that physicians' examination skills have deteriorated over the years. While advances in technology, including laboratory testing and radiologic imaging, are partly to blame for this decline, clinical skills training during medical school and residency are also factors. According to Dr. Sal Mangione, Director of the Physical Diagnosis Curriculum at Jefferson Medical

College, too little time is spent during medical school learning these skills. "Surveys have indicated that less than 16% of attending time may be spent at the patient's side."[18]

Physical exam skills have important, obvious ramifications for patient care, and the education you receive in this area during medical school is critical. If you don't learn certain skills at this stage of your education, you may never have the opportunity to do so. In one study, researchers observed interns and residents, and noted frequent errors in physical exam technique.[19] Errors included improper manual technique or use of instruments. The authors asserted that these errors resulted from a failure to learn the necessary psychomotor skills during the preclinical years.

In the real world of medicine, these deficiencies in skills have serious consequences. In a study of interns and residents on a general medicine service, at least one serious physical exam error was made for nearly two-thirds of the patients examined. The errors included failure to detect splenomegaly or focal neurological signs, findings that once discovered led to significant changes in diagnosis and treatment.[20]

While clinical courses such as "Introduction to Clinical Medicine" and "Physical Diagnosis" teach these skills, this is one area where students cannot rely on passive learning. In Chapter 6, you'll learn how to make the most of your physical exam education. These skills aren't easy to learn. While a recent study showed that third-year med students felt quite confident about their ability to measure blood pressure, students were significantly less confident in their ability to assess retinal vasculature, detect a thyroid nodule, or measure jugular venous pressure.[21]

You'll also learn the importance of soliciting preceptor feedback. If errors aren't picked up at this stage of your education, they may never be. While you might expect that your future residents or attendings would be able to correct your performance, the literature has shown that students on clerkships often aren't observed while performing physical exams. They are typically assumed to already possess the necessary skills.

The chapter also addresses other facets of physical exams, including the patient's comfort. You'll learn how to approach an often uncomfortable situation in a manner that most reassures the patient. In the article "Learning to Doctor," Conrad aptly describes the concerns of students:[22]

Students tell patients twice their age to get undressed, and then cross conventional barriers of interpersonal space to inspect the intimacies of their bodies. In addition to anxiety about doing it right, students frequently must deal with their own reactions to their patient as well as discomforting feelings of being invasive.

Research

In a presentation to medical students titled "Research in Medical School," Dr. Daniel West discussed reasons why students should consider involvement in research. Dr. West noted that participation in research allows medical students to explore a specialty in more depth, enhance critical thinking and other related skills, assess suitability for a career in academic medicine, and strengthen credentials for residency positions.[23] Medical students recognize these benefits as well. In a survey of students at three medical schools, 83% agreed that participation in research was valuable within their medical education.[24]

In Chapter 7, we'll discuss these benefits in more depth. There are significant benefits to participation in research, and while barriers exist, many medical students are able to overcome these barriers, enhance their own skills and education, and make contributions to the scientific literature.

Research training leads to better critical thinking skills. The ability to critically appraise the literature is essential to the practice of evidence-based medicine. The University of Arizona College of Medicine writes that "as future physicians, being able to critically read a scientific journal along with keeping abreast of new medical innovations is an important facet of practice that can profoundly impact patient outcomes."[25] In a recent article, Mayo researchers wrote about how research benefits medical students.[26] "Studies have shown that students who had conducted research during medical school reported gains in knowledge and skills in appraising the literature, analyzing data, and writing for publication, along with more positive attitudes toward future research." Students report significant benefits from learning the process of research, from conception of an idea to publication and presentation. It is important for all physicians to learn about literature review, hypothesis generation, study methodology, and data analysis.

Research also has known benefits in the residency selection process. Dr. Scott Pretorius, former Radiology Residency Program Director at the University of Pennsylvania, wrote that "in this competitive market for radiology residency slots, medical students with research backgrounds...allow themselves the opportunity to stand out in a field of increasingly highly qualified applicants. As an advisor of medical students, I routinely recommend that students intending to apply for radiology residency seek out a research mentor and undertake some kind of research project."[27] In a survey of University of Tennessee medical students, 63% reported that research experience was beneficial in helping them secure a residency position.[28]

As you're applying for residency positions, it's important to know your competition. Among dermatology applicants, nearly 95% had participated in at least one research project, with over 80% claiming at least one abstract, publication, or presentation.[29] In radiation oncology, among U.S. senior applicants, only 9 of the 152 applicants reported not having a single abstract, publication, or presentation. While it's not a prerequisite for students applying to competitive fields, a student may stand out due to their lack of any research experience in these fields.

While students recognize the benefits of research, many find the barriers to involvement daunting. Difficulty finding a research supervisor can be a significant barrier, with only 44% of students in one study reporting that it was easy to identify one.[24] In this chapter, you'll learn how to identify research opportunities at your institution. We highlight ways to identify the "right" research mentor, as well as what to discuss with potential mentors and how to evaluate potential research projects.

In evaluating research experience during medical school, residency programs will look closely at the level of your involvement. Did you merely collect data? Or were you involved through all phases of the project (design of the project, data collection, analysis of the data, and writing the manuscript)? Programs also assess your productivity. Did your work result in a tangible measure, such as an abstract, manuscript, or presentation at a meeting? For many students involved in research, a publication or presentation resulting from their work would be ideal. While this isn't always possible, in this chapter you'll learn how to approach the issue of publication and learn about journals that are targeted to medical students.

You'll also learn about possibilities for presentation, even if those opportunities aren't initiated by your research mentor. Students may seek out opportunities to present their work at local, regional, national, and international meetings. At Stanford University School of Medicine, 52% of medical students had presented at a national meeting.[30] Symposiums and meetings geared to medical student research presentations include the National Student Research Forum (NSRF), Eastern-Atlantic Student Research Forum (ESRF), and Western Student Medical Research Forum (WSMRF). The NSRF is held at the University of Texas Medical Branch in Galveston, and provides a forum for students to give either poster or oral presentations.[31] Over 30 awards are given at this annual event.

Time has been reported as a major barrier to pursuing research in medical school. Many students become involved in research in the summer between the first and second years of medical school. Opportunities for summer research may also be available for newly admitted students who haven't yet started medical school. At the Mt. Sinai School of Medicine, 54 to 65% of students participated in summer research between 2001 and 2004.[32]

Some students are interested in a more substantial research experience, and in this chapter you'll learn about some of the "year-out" opportunities available to students across the country. The Clinical Research Fellowship for Medical Students, sponsored by the Doris Duke Charitable Foundation, offers one-year fellowships at one of 12 selected institutions in the U.S. The HHMI – NIH (Howard Hughes Medical Institute - National Institutes of Health) Research Scholars Program and NIH Clinical Research Training Program allow participants the opportunity to work on the NIH campus. Research Training Fellowships through the HHMI are also available to students, and support one year of research at a variety of academic institutions. This chapter highlights a number of other opportunities that are available for students interested in more substantial research experience.

Extracurricular Activities

As in college, the learning environment in medical school extends beyond the classroom, and institutions offer valuable opportunities to participate in a variety of extracurricular activities. For example, at the Case Western Reserve University, there are over 40 medical student organizations.[33]

Involvement in these organizations provides a number of opportunities and benefits, and in Chapter 8 you'll learn more about the opportunities available. One of the most important is the further development of skills that are directly applicable to success as a physician. A few examples of vital skills in the daily life of a physician are teamwork, self-discipline, time management, and leadership, all of which are strengthened outside of the classroom through extracurricular involvement. Involvement in organizations is a way to develop and strengthen bonds with classmates, and since student organizations often have a faculty advisor or sponsor, students have extraordinary opportunities to work closely with faculty members. Such opportunities are usually unavailable to students during the preclinical years.

Some students are awarded recognition for their involvement. Every year, the American Medical Association honors 15 students with

AMA Foundation Leadership Awards. These awards recognize students who have demonstrated "strong, nonclinical leadership skills in advocacy, community service, public health, and/or education."[34] Many other organizations recognize student involvement as well. When evaluating a student's contributions, organizations seek evidence of leadership, commitment, and the ability to make meaningful contributions to the goals of an organization. Some students, after reviewing the opportunities available at their school, commit to starting a new organization or founding a new chapter of a national organization. In this chapter, you'll learn what questions to ask, and what resources are available, as you review your opportunities.

Involvement may also help students reach their professional goals. Extracurricular activities "might provide evidence for non-cognitive attributes that predict success," writes Dr. Andrew Lee, Chairman of the Department of Ophthalmology at The Methodist Hospital.[35] "Leadership skills demonstrated by being an officer in extracurricular activities or being an Eagle Scout, or a leader or founder of a new organization or club are all looked upon favorably. The second goal is to look for evidence of non-cognitive attributes that might make a superior ophthalmologist (conflict resolution, team work, leadership ability, communication skills, performance under stress, maturity, seriousness of purpose, prior scholarly activity). Finally, programs are looking to graduate (and thus select) residents who will make the program proud."

In fact, extracurricular activities do serve as a significant nonacademic factor in the residency selection process. In a recent NRMP survey of 1,840 program directors representing the nineteen largest medical specialties, 59% of respondents cited volunteer/extracurricular experiences as a factor in selecting applicants to interview.[36]

Evidence suggests that meaningful contributions in extracurricular activities, particularly leadership, may serve as a predictor of residency performance. In one study of emergency medicine residency program directors, having a "distinctive factor" such as being a championship athlete or medical school officer, was one of three factors most predictive of residency performance.[37] In a study to determine predictors of otolaryngology resident success using data available at the time of interview, candidates having an exceptional trait such as leadership experience were found to be rated higher as residents.[38]

Community Service

In researching community service opportunities for medical students, we found ourselves amazed and inspired by the accomplishments of medical schools, medical school organizations, and individual medical students. In Chapter 9, you'll hear about the significant contributions made by students. You'll learn about opportunities for participation in community service, the impact your participation can have on the health of the community, and how your involvement can help you grow personally and professionally.

According to Dr. Aaron McGuffin, Senior Associate Dean for Medical Education at Marshall University School of Medicine, "there has been 2,700 hours of community service donated from the medical school students in the past 12 months. That is a lot of time in addition to doing their medical school work."[39] In 2008, the AAMC found that a significant percentage of medical school applicants had been involved in community service.[40] Sixty-three percent of the applicants reported nonmedical volunteer experience, while medical volunteer experience was reported by 77% of applicants. "They have a real sense of service, commitment, and discovery that I know we all want in a future doctor at our bedside," said Dr. Darrell Kirch, the AAMC President.[41]

While the provision of community service has been a major area of emphasis at U.S. medical schools for years, educators have recently stressed the importance of fostering education in community service among medical students. In 1998, Seifer defined service learning as "a structured learning experience that combines community service with preparation and reflection."[42] The Liaison Committee on Medical Education (LCME), which is responsible for the accreditation of medical schools, recommends that schools should not only provide students with sufficient opportunities "to participate in service-learning activities," but also "encourage and support student participation."[43]

Many schools provide such opportunities for service learning. In 2001, the Morehouse School of Medicine established the Center for Community Health and Service - Learning to engage students and other healthcare professionals in community service and service learning. Partnering with other organizations in the Atlanta area, the center aims to address the health disparities affecting underserved populations. At the University of New Mexico School of Medicine, community service is a key priority.[44] Educators have gone beyond just encouragement by freeing students in the afternoons during the first year for service engagement.

At other schools, student organizations have been able to make significant contributions to their communities. The AAMC's Medicine in the Community Grant Program (formerly known as Caring for Community) offers grant awards to medical students who wish to initiate, develop, and run a community service project.[45] According to the AAMC, "Medicine in the Community will help students to translate great ideas into meaningful service by contributing needed start-up and supplemental funds." Past recipients of the grant include the Medical College of Wisconsin Hmong Health Education Program. HHEP is an effort to improve health education and healthcare services for Wisconsin's Hmong population through educational workshops, outreach programs, support groups, and public service announcements. Another past recipient is the University of New Mexico School of Medicine Community Vision Project. Through the use of mobile eye clinics, basic vision care services are provided to American Indian and Hispanic populations.

For students wishing to make significant contributions to their communities, a number of organizations provide grants and assistance. In this chapter, you'll learn about grants and resources available to students who wish to initiate their own service project, as well as hear about other successful projects. For example, the Medical Student Section of the AMA (AMA-MSS) has created a list and description of projects that AMA-MSS chapters across the country have developed and implemented.[46] Since the 1970s, *Project Bank: The Encyclopedia of Public Health and Community Projects*, a tool offered by the AMA Alliance, has served as a useful compendium of community service projects conducted by state and county Alliances.[47]

Student-run health clinics have been initiated at many medical schools, and such involvement can have a significant impact on the personal and professional growth of medical students. At the University of California Davis, 85% of medical students volunteer in student clinics during their tenure in medical school.[48] "Students are often changed in unexpected, profound, and lasting ways after experiencing firsthand healthcare delivery to the poor, underserved, and marginalized," explains Dr. Ed Farrell, a physician volunteer at the Stout Street Clinic, which is run by students attending the University of Colorado School of Medicine.[49]

Not all schools have initiated such clinics. For motivated students, a number of resources are available for those wishing to establish a student-run health clinic. In an article published in JAMA, Cohen wrote "Eight Steps for Starting a Student-Run Clinic."[50] Another useful resource, "25 Steps to Starting a Student-Run Clinic," is available at the Society of Student-Run Free Clinics website.[51]

Community service provides known benefits to students as well. Research has shown that volunteering increases positive feelings, improves mental health, reduces the risk of depression, and lowers stress levels.[52-54] Participation may also improve communication skills, a vital skill in medicine. Community service is also a significant nonacademic factor in the residency selection process. Once accepted for an interview, the depth and breadth of your involvement in community service may help you stand out in a sea of academically qualified applicants.

Mentoring

The further we've progressed in our own careers, the more it becomes apparent how many individuals have helped us along the way. To achieve professional success in almost any field requires help. This may not be initially obvious to medical students, who are used to studying hard and achieving high grades on their own. Reaching medical school though, definitely required help. Professors who provided help outside of the classroom, researchers who offered the opportunity to participate in their project, advisors who provided letters of recommendation: the list goes on.

Succeeding in medical school, and succeeding in the residency match itself, requires even more assistance. At this next stage of your career, informed guidance and advice becomes even more important. For more competitive specialties or programs, you'll also require additional qualifications, which may mean approaching faculty members for research opportunities, in addition to the critically important letters of recommendation.

The definition of a mentor is one who "takes a special interest in helping another person develop into a successful professional."[55] Information, advice, and guidance from a knowledgeable faculty member is invaluable, and has the potential to impact your career in significant ways.

Sometimes the hardest part of initiating an effective relationship is just knowing how to get started. You'll be approaching respected, accomplished, busy individuals, and it can be difficult to know how to approach faculty members without appearing intrusive or presumptuous. For most students, asking for help from individuals in a position of authority can be intimidating. As a preclinical student, you also may have had limited experience in dealing with faculty on an individual level, and knowing what's acceptable can be hard to determine. Therefore, we provide advice from faculty experienced in this area. Certain approaches would be considered acceptable and non-intrusive by most faculty.

Some medical schools have formal mentoring programs. If such a program doesn't exist at your school, then you'll need confidence and possibly persistence to initiate a relationship. In one study, 28% of students met their mentors during inpatient clerkships, 19% through research activities, and 9% during outpatient clerkships.[56]

Local, regional, and state medical societies may have established mentoring programs. For example, the Santa Clara County Medical Association has a Mentor Program for Stanford medical students.[57] National organizations are committed to mentoring future doctors also.   The Society of Academic Emergency Medicine (SAEM) has a medical student virtual advisor program open to students at all institutions.[58] Through this program, students can query experienced individuals about a variety of issues, including the EM residency application process. Dr. Joshua Grossman reminds students that mentors don't have to be in close proximity to you. "Your mentor does not need to be someone involved with your residency program that you see on a daily basis. By sharing your experience with someone removed from the situation you may be able to gain a different and beneficial perspective.[59]

While many of us have worked with assigned advisors during our education, a mentoring relationship is unique, and can be hard to delineate. In Chapter 10, you'll hear from mentors and organizations about the best way to develop such a relationship, and specifics on expectations and etiquette. The Association of Women Surgeons writes "A mentor is a unique individual to you: neither friend, nor colleague, but something of a combination of these and more. Because the relationship differs from those you have with others in your department, you may feel more relaxed and less constrained by professional protocol. This is acceptable to a point, but make certain that you respect the relationship."[60]

What do students talk about with a mentor? Issues may include those related to specialty choice, career satisfaction, wellness, work/life balance, residency selection process, research, interpersonal skills, professionalism, ethics, and courses. Once they have a firm idea of career choice, many students schedule meetings to discuss match strategy, seeking advice on steps they can take at their level to establish their credentials and strengthen their applications.

It can be intimidating and challenging to seek advice from qualified, well-informed faculty members. Is it worth seeking a mentor? While mentors can prove helpful throughout medical school, they can provide invaluable guidance during the process of preparing for the residency match. In researching our companion book, *The Successful Match: 200 Rules to Succeed in the Residency Match*, we asked applicants what they found most difficult about the residency application process. A number of applicants commented on the same issue. "There's so much conflicting information out there. How do you know what to believe? Who should you listen to?" Applicants with mentors have a decided advantage. Students benefit greatly when the wisdom, experience, and perspective of a knowledgeable faculty member are used to help them. Having a mentor to guide you through the complex residency application process is recognized by students as an important factor in boosting the strength of their application.

Well-being

In the past, issues of medical student well-being weren't a priority. Today, though, medical educators recognize that the intense pressures of medical school can have serious consequences for a medical student's physical health and emotional well-being. Research has demonstrated that these aren't just soft issues; they have real ramifications for patient care as well. In a recent study of pediatric residents, 20% of participants met criteria for depression, and these residents made over six times as many medication errors as their non-depressed colleagues.[61]

It's clear that medical school can be intensely stressful. In a survey of medical students, Wolf asked students to rate medical school stressors on a scale of 1 (not stressful) to 7 (extremely stressful).[62] The top four stressors, out of 16 ranked, were examinations, amount of classwork, financial responsibilities, and lack of time for recreation and entertainment. In a survey of medical students at 16 U.S. schools, 60% of first-year students reported either "moderate" or "a lot" of stress in the last two weeks.[63] This stress can lead to physician burnout, a condition which is characterized by emotional depletion from one's work, depersonalization, and the perception that one's work is inconsequential. In a survey of medical students in Minnesota, 45% had burnout.[64]

We chose to emphasize issues of medical student well-being within this chapter for several reasons. One was to highlight the impact of med school stressors on a student's health and well-being. Evidence indicates that this impact can be significant, and it is common for medical students to be affected. Even more importantly, in this chapter you'll learn how to buffer this stress. You'll learn about effective coping strategies identified by researchers. There is significant evidence that sleep, exercise, and the maintenance of strong social connections can provide strong buffers against the stressors of med school. Many students let these activities go first, though, in their efforts to focus on coursework and exams. However, studies indicate that these strategies, and others, should actually be priorities at times of intense stress. In a cross-sectional study of medical students, approximately 77% suffered some degree of anxiety.[65] Anxiety symptoms were considerably less common in students exercising at least 30 minutes three times a week. Another study revealed that "strong social ties was the factor most positively related to better health and life satisfaction" among a group of first-year medical students.[66]

It's important to develop effective coping strategies during the preclinical years, as the clinical care of patients only adds to stress. Dr. Liselotte Dyrbye, a faculty member at the Mayo Clinic, has performed extensive research in this area. She states that medical students need to have "the skills necessary to assess personal distress, determine its effects on their care of patients, recognize when they need assistance, and develop strategies to promote their own well-being. These skills are essential to maintain perspective, professionalism, and resilience through the course of a career..."[64]

In this chapter, you'll learn more about coping strategies. One effective strategy is problem-focused coping, in which efforts are made to solve or manage the problem causing the distress. Emotion-focused coping is another effective strategy, among many others. As a new med student, it's helpful to learn about how you cope with issues. In 1997, Charles Carver, a professor at the University of Miami, developed the brief COPE questionnaire, which can be used as a tool to help determine the coping strategies that you tend to use.[67] If your total scores are higher in the coping strategy categories of self-distraction, denial, substance abuse, or self-blame, you'll need to learn how to develop and use healthier and more effective coping skills. Dr. Julie Gentile, Director of Medical Student Mental Health Services at the Boonshoft School of Medicine at Wright State University, states that medical school "is a critical period in which to develop and utilize functional and effective coping strategies"[68]

Professionalism

What is professionalism, and why does it matter?

Consider the following observation made by a student:

Two doctors were down the hall from each other, and there were people around. One said to the other, "Did you hear about Mr. X?" And the other doctor said no, and he made a face like a dead face...sticking his tongue out, crossing his eyes, and tilting his head to the side. If anybody had noticed they wouldn't have been too happy with it.[69]

Students must be prepared to deal with issues of professionalism in their peers, in members of the healthcare team, and even in their teachers. Researchers found that exposure to unprofessional behavior began early in the medical education process and increased in each successive year. In Year 1 of medical school, 66% of students had "heard derogatory comments not in patient's presence" and 35% had "observed unethical conduct by residents or attending physicians."[70]

Why else does professionalism matter?

The vast majority of the students we meet have core values and a strong sense of personal integrity. Many therefore assume that issues of professionalism, while they may impact others around them, don't have any relevance to their own behavior. This is due to the common assumption that our core values regarding unethical behavior are stable over time. Studies of medical students contradict this assumption.

In one study, medical students were given a list of 11 unprofessional behaviors, and asked "Is the following behavior unprofessional for a medical student?"[71] Students were surveyed before matriculation and again six months into their first year of medical school. Researchers found that behaviors originally considered unprofessional rapidly became more acceptable. Medical students were also presented with four different scenarios, and asked "Must one do the following to be professional?" For the scenario "Report Cheating to a Professor or Administrator," 69% of students originally answered "yes." Six months into medical school, only 41% answered "yes."

There are therefore two core reasons to focus on this field. If you're a medical student, you are likely to witness lapses in professionalism in patient care, and you need to be prepared to deal with those lapses and protect your patients. You also need to define and protect your own core values and personal integrity.

What is professionalism? The foundation of the medical profession rests upon the trust that patients place in their physicians. Professionalism focuses on this foundation of trust. Although it's been defined in various ways, the core values and elements agreed upon include honesty, integrity, compassion, empathy, ability to communicate effectively with patients, and respect for others. Professionalism is a hot topic in undergraduate medical education. A number of medical education organizations, including the American Board of Internal Medicine, the Association of American Medical Colleges, and the National Board of Medical Examiners, have established professionalism as a required competency across the spectrum of medical education.

Medical schools, in turn, have made it a point to educate preclinical students.

Many students, when hearing about a curriculum on professionalism, have similar reactions. "I already hold these values. Why should any of this concern me?" The studies that we describe in this chapter provide a definitive answer to that question. Most students are surprised to learn that the stresses and challenges of medical school can affect attitude, behavior, and conduct. However, this conclusion is clearly supported by a number of studies.

Even though medical students may actually harm patients when they act unethically, such actions persist. In a survey of students at a single medical school, 13 to 24% admitted to cheating during the clinical years of medical school.[72] Examples included "recording tasks not performed" and "lying about having ordered tests." In another study, students were asked whether they had heard of or witnessed unethical behaviors on the part of their student colleagues.[73] In response, 21% had personal knowledge of students "reporting a pelvic examination as 'normal' during rounds when it had been inadvertently omitted from the physical examination."

As students, you are likely to witness lapses in professional behavior, and may witness outright unethical behavior and fraud. These issues affect every level of our profession, and therefore you have to be prepared. You must guard against lapses in your own behavior, and be prepared to deal with lapses in colleagues or supervisors. As physicians, our goal is to treat and protect the patient, and this can be challenging in the real world of clinical medicine.

In a survey, third-year students at the University of Texas Medical Branch at Galveston were asked to evaluate their physicians' professionalism.[74] Although this review of nearly 3,000 evaluation forms revealed significant praise for positive faculty role modeling, negative comments were not infrequent. The majority dealt with "issues of language use, inappropriate use of humor, disrespectful treatment of patients or colleagues, and apparent disinterest in teaching."

Although we think of physicians as highly compassionate and ethical individuals, ethical lapses can extend to the highest levels of our profession. In a stunning case of scientific fraud, Dr. Scott Reuben, a highly regarded anesthesiologist whose research has significantly impacted how physicians treat surgical patients for pain, was found to have fabricated results in over 20 published studies.[75] In some cases, he is alleged to have even invented patients.

Choosing a Specialty

For many students, having just arrived at med school and facing voluminous amounts of material to be learned and retained, the focus will be on just making it through. Why, then, have we devoted a large chapter to the topic of choosing and exploring a specialty?

Those medical students who are able to plan and strategize for the residency match have a decided advantage. For the most competitive specialties, great grades and high USMLE scores are not enough. You'll need great letters of recommendation and support from faculty advocates. You'll also need additional distinctions. Most applicants to the competitive specialties will have performed research, and many will have publications or presentations to their name. Some programs look for additional factors of distinction, such as involvement in extracurricular activities, evidence of leadership, and commitment to service.

We present this information not to scare you, but to prepare you. These are the realities of the residency match today, and students who are prepared for these realities have a definite advantage. Your preparation doesn't need to be an overwhelming experience, either. It can start with the basics, such as exploring different specialties by shadowing faculty or speaking to residents. You may choose to take an aptitude test to help guide you in your exploration of specialties. Many students maximize their free summer after first year by participating in research. Those who are knowledgeable can obtain research grants from organizations to fund their research. This has tangible benefits. It results in research experience, an awarded research grant, and the opportunity to develop a relationship with a research mentor who may be able to support your application down the road.

In this chapter, you'll learn more about how to approach the process of choosing a specialty. You'll learn how to approach your target department, and how to cultivate opportunities. You'll gain from the insider knowledge presented in this section, as the chapter outlines, for each and every specialty, detailed specifics about medical student opportunities. These include mentorship programs, research grants targeted to medical students, and information about national meetings.

Why is it important to at least start thinking about your specialty choice now? While many med students wait until the clinical years to assess fit, this approach can be problematic. At most schools, students are required to rotate through the major or core specialties (internal medicine, general surgery, pediatrics, psychiatry, family medicine, obstetrics & gynecology) before pursuing clerkships in other fields. After completing these core rotations during the third year, students aren't left with much time. Most have two to three months of elective time to explore other specialties before they need to decide, since residency applications are typically submitted in September of the fourth year. For example, in a survey of med schools, it was found that anesthesiology is an elective rotation in 66% of schools.[76] For most students, this means that unless you attend a school with a flexible clerkship curriculum, you won't be able to rotate through the specialty until the beginning of your fourth year.

This can have a decided impact on a student's career. In one study of medical students, 26.2% were unsure of their specialty choice at matriculation.[77] Surprisingly, a similar proportion remained undecided at graduation. According to Gwen Garrison, Director of Student and Applicant Services at the AAMC, 30% of residents "either switch from their intended specialty after a transitional or preliminary year or switch outright during their specialty residency."[78] Dr. George Blackall, Director of Student Development at Penn State University College of Medicine, offers some reasons why residents switch. "Residents primarily switch because they a) realize their initial choice is not as interesting as another specialty, or b) desire a different lifestyle, level of flexibility, or income."[78]

In this chapter, you'll learn how to start the process of exploring a specialty. During the preclinical years, one way to assess fit for specialties is by completing personality-type inventories. The premise of this approach is that people are most satisfied professionally when there is a good match between their specialty choice and their values, skills, and interests. Commonly used assessment methods include the AAMC Careers in Medicine program and the Glaxo Wellcome Pathway Evaluation Program. The AAMC Careers in Medicine (CiM) is a structured program designed to help students gain a better understanding of their personality, values, skills, and interests. The program also allows for exploration of different specialties. The AAMC writes that "as you work through the CiM program, you'll gain the tools to make an informed decision, based on guided self-reflection and the information you'll gather about many career options available to you."[79] Another resource is the Medical Specialty Aptitude Test, an online test developed by the University of Virginia School of Medicine.[80] It is based on content and material from the book, How to Choose a Medical Specialty, by Anita Taylor. The website indicates that "you will be asked to rate your tendencies compared to the tendencies of physicians in each specialty. The higher your score for a given specialty, the more similar you are to the physicians in that specialty."

What is the most important factor in choosing a specialty? In a recent survey of graduating medical students, approximately 97%

reported that fit with personality, skills, and interests was moderately or strongly influential in choosing which specialty to pursue as a career.[81] No other factor was given as much importance.

For many students, work/life balance also plays an important role. In the 2010 AAMC Medical School Graduation Questionnaire, over 11,000 graduating students were asked, "How influential was work/life balance in helping you choose your specialty?"[81] Over 70% of respondents reported work/life balance as being either moderately or strongly influential in their decision-making process. In 1989, Schwartz introduced the term controllable lifestyle to refer to "specialties that offer regular and predictable hours."[82] These specialties are often characterized by fewer hours spent at work and less frequent on-call duties, allowing for greater personal time and flexibility to pursue other activities. Specialties that are generally felt to offer a controllable lifestyle include anesthesiology, dermatology, neurology, ophthalmology, otolaryngology, pathology, psychiatry, and radiology.

Research has shown that efforts to explore specialties during the preclinical years can increase the certainty of specialty choice.[83] In this chapter, you'll learn about multiple avenues to learn more about specialties during the preclinical years. Examples include:

- Identify and work with a mentor
- Volunteer for clinical experiences (e.g., shadowing)
- Perform specialty-specific research
- Meet and speak with as many physicians as you can in your specialties of interest
- Attend local and national specialty organization meetings
- Join specialty interest groups (e.g., Internal Medicine Interest Group, Emergency Medicine Interest Group)

For each of these avenues, we've included specifics on how to proceed. Medical students value mentoring relationships, but identifying and working with a faculty member can be difficult. According to Dr. Gus Garmel, Co-Program Director of the Stanford-Kaiser Emergency Medicine Residency Program, finding a mentor is not easy.[84] "How students find faculty mentors is challenging, because their exposure to a broad selection of emergency medicine faculty may be limited early in their training." We've provided suggestions on how to proceed for each of the specialties. For example, the American College of Physicians (ACP) has created a Mentoring Database. To access the database, which includes program directors, clerkship directors, chairs of medicine, practicing internists, and residents, you must be a member. Mentors are available to answer "specific questions about scheduling your summer preceptorships, getting through the match, and preparing for clerkships and residency interviews…"[85]

We've also included further information about identifying research opportunities. For many of the most competitive specialties, such as dermatology and radiation oncology, your competition will almost all have performed research. Therefore, if you're considering dermatology as a career, you may wish to participate in research between the first and second years of medical school. Research experience has significant educational benefits. Beyond those benefits, research allows a student the chance to develop a relationship with their research supervisor.

In this chapter, you'll gain from the insider knowledge presented for each and every specialty, with detailed, specific information about medical student opportunities.

Chapter excerpted from the book - Success in Medical School: Insider Advice for the Preclinical Years

References

[1]Klatt E, Klatt C. How much is too much reading for medical students? Assigned reading and reading rates at one medical school. *Acad Med* 2011; 86(9): 1079-83.

[2]West C, Sadoski M. Do study strategies predict academic performance in medical school? *Med Educ* 2011; 45(7): 696-703.

[3]Collins G, Cassie J, Daggett C. The role of the attending physician in clinical training. *J Med Educ* 1978; 53: 429-31.

[4]University of Alabama Birmingham School of Medicine. Advice from MS-2 Students. Available at: http://main.uab.edu/uasom/2/show.asp?durki=111766. Accessed October 22, 2011.

[5]Finnerty E, Chauvin S, Bonamino G, Andrews M, Carroll R, Pangaro L. Flexner revisited: the role and value of the basic sciences in medical education. *Acad Med* 2010; 85 (2): 349-55.

[6]Green M, Jones P, Thomas J. Selection criteria for residency: results of a national program directors survey. *Acad Med* 2009; 84(3): 362-7.

[7]Medscape. The USMLE: Ten Questions. Available at: http://www.medscape.com/viewarticle/403686. Accessed October 19, 2011.

[8]NBME. Available at: http://www.nbme.org. Accessed October 29, 2011.

[9]University of Utah School of Medicine. Preparing for Step 1. Available at: medicine.utah.edu/learningresources/usmle/step1.htm. Accessed October 19, 2011.

[10]University of California San Francisco School of Medicine. Rx for Success on STEP 1 of The Boards. Available at: http://medschool.ucsf.edu/medstudents/documents/step1success.pdf. Accessed October 19, 2011.

[11]NBOME. Available at: http://www.nbome.org. Accessed November 4, 2011.

[12]NRMP. Available at: http://www.nrmp.org. Accessed September 12, 2011.

[13]Cummings M, Sefcik D. The impact of osteopathic physicians' participation in ACGME-accredited postdoctoral programs, 1985-2006. *Acad Med* 2009; 84(6): 733-6.

[14]Moss F, McManus I. The anxieties of new clinical students. *Med Educ* 1992; 26: 17-20.

[15]O'Brien B, Cooke M, Irby D. Perceptions and attributions of third-year student struggles in clerkships: do students and clerkship directors agree? *Acad Med* 2007; 82(10): 970-978.

[16]Windish D, Paulman P, Goroll A, Bass E. Do clerkship directors think medical students are prepared for the clerkship years? *Acad Med* 2004; 79(1): 56-61.

[17]Hauer K, Teherani A, Kerr K, O'Sullivan P, Irby, D. Student performance problems in medical school clinical skills assessments. *Acad Med* 2007; 82(10): S69-S72.

[18]ACP Internist. Good diagnostic skills should begin at the bedside. Available at: http://www.acpinternist.org/archives/2001/02/diagnostics.htm. Accessed February 1, 2012.

[19]Wiener S, Nathanson M. Physical examination: frequently observed errors. *JAMA* 1976; 236(7): 852-5.

[20]Wray N, Friedland J. Detection and correction of house staff error in physical diagnosis. *JAMA* 1983; 249: 1035-7.

[21]Wu E, Fagan M, Reinert S, Diaz J. Self-confidence in and perceived utility of the physical examination: a comparison of medical students, residents, and faculty internists. *J Gen Intern Med* 2007; 22(12): 1725-30.

[22]Conrad P. Learning to doctor: reflections on recent accounts of the medical school years. *Journal of Health and Social Behavior* 1988; 29(4): 323-32.

[23]University of California Davis School of Medicine. Available at: http://mdscholars.ucdavis.edu/Research%20in%20Medical%20School.ppt. Accessed February 9, 2012.

[24]Siemens D, Punnen S, Wong J, Kanji N. A survey on the attitudes towards research in medical school. *BMC Med Educ* 2010; 22: 10: 4.

[25]University of Arizona Medical Student Research Program. Available at: http://www.msrp.medicine.arizona.edu/dist_guidrat.htm. Accessed February 9, 2012.

[26]Dyrbye L, Davidson L, Cook D. Publications and presentations resulting from required research by students at Mayo Medical School, 1976-2003. *Acad Med* 2008; 83(6): 604-10.

[27]Pretorius E. Medical student research: a residency director's perspective. *Acad Radiol* 2002; 9(7): 808-9.

[28]Solomon S, Tom S, Pichert J, Wasserman D, Powers A. Impact of medical student research in the development of physician scientists. *J Investig Med* 2002; 51(3): 149-56.

[29]National Resident Match Program Charting Outcomes in the Match. www.nrmp.org. Accessed August 1, 2010.

[30]Jacobs C, Cross P. The value of medical student research: the experience at Stanford University School of Medicine. *Med Educ* 1995; 29(5): 342-6.

[31]National Student Research Forum. Available at: http://www.utmb.edu/nsrf/. Accessed February 9, 2012.

[32]Zier K, Friedman E, Smith L. Supportive programs increase medical students' research interest and productivity. *J Investig Med* 2006; 54(4): 201-7.

[33]Case Western Reserve University School of Medicine. Available at: http://casemed.case.edu/. Accessed February 12, 2012.

[34]American Medical Association. Available at: http://www.ama-assn.org/ama/pub/about-ama/ama-foundation/our-programs/public-health/excellence-medicine-awards.page. Accessed February 12, 2012.

[35]The Successful Match: Getting into Ophthalmology. Available at: http://studentdoctor.net/2009/08/the-successful-match-interview-with-dr-andrew-lee-ophthalmology/. Accessed February 12, 2012.

[36]NRMP 2010 Program Director Survey. Available at: http://www.nrmp.org/data/index.html. Accessed February 12, 2012.

[37]Hayden S, Hayden M, Garnst A. What characteristics of applicants to emergency medicine residency programs predict future success as an emergency medicine resident. *Acad Emerg Med* 2005; 12(3): 206-10.

[38]Daly K, Levine S, Adams G. Predictors for resident success in otolaryngology. *J Am Coll Surg* 2006; 202 (4): 649-54.

[39]Joan C. Edwards School of Medicine at Marshall University. Available at: http://www.marshallparthenon.com/news/med-students-earning-cash-for-community-service-1.1936252. Accessed September 12, 2011.
[40]Association of American Medical Colleges. Available at: http://www.aamc.org/newsroom/pressrel/2008/enrollmentdata2008.pdf. Accessed July 23, 2011.
[41]American Academy of Family Physicians. Available at: http://www.aafp.org/online/en/home/publications/news/news-now/resident-student-focus/20081119med-school-enroll.html. Accessed February 12, 2012.
[42]Seifer SD. Service-learning: community-campus partnerships for health professions education. *Acad Med* 1998; 73(3): 273-7.
[43]Liaison Committee on Medical Education (LCME) Available at: http://www.lcme.org/standard.htm#servicelearning. Accessed February 12, 2012.
[44]University of New Mexico School of Medicine. Available at: http://hsc.unm.edu/som/. Accessed February 22, 2012.
[45]AAMC Medicine in the Community Grant Program. Available at: http://www.aamc.org/about/awards/cfc/start.htm. Accessed February 12, 2012.
[46]American Medical Association Medical Student Section. Available at: http://www.ama-assn.org. Accessed February 12, 2012.
[47]AMA Alliance Project Bank. Available at: http://www.amaalliance.org/site/epage/40331_625.htm. Accessed February 12, 2012.
[48]University of California Davis School of Medicine. Available at: http://www-med.ucdavis.edu/. Accessed September 12, 2011.
[49]American Medical Association Virtual Mentor. Available at: http://virtualmentor.ama-assn.org/2005/07/medu1-0507.html. Accessed February 12, 2012.
[50]Cohen J. Eight Steps for starting a student-run clinic. *JAMA* 1995; 273: 434–5.
[51]Society of Student-Run Free Clinics. Available at: http://www.studentrunfreeclinics.org/index.php?option=com_content&view=article&id=65&Itemid=144. Accessed February 12, 2012.
[52]Thoits P, Hewitt L. Volunteer work and well-being. *Journal of Health and Social Behavior* 2001; 42(2): 115-31.
[53]Van Willigen M. Differential benefits of volunteering across the life course. *The Journals of Gerontology Series B: Psychological Sciences and Social Sciences* 2000; 55B(5): S308-S318.
[54]Rietschlin J. Voluntary association membership and psychological distress. *J Health Soc Behav* 1998; 39; 348-55.
[55]Adviser, teacher, role model, friend. Available at: http://stills.nap.edu/readingroom/books/mentor. Accessed March 13, 2008. Washington, DC: National Academy Press; 1997.
[56]Aagaard E, Hauer K. A cross-sectional descriptive study of mentoring relationships formed by medical students. *J Gen Intern Med* 2003; 18: 298-302.
[57]Santa Clara County Medical Association Mentor Program for Stanford medical students. Available at: http://med.stanford.edu/mentors/. Accessed February 9, 2012.

[58]Society of Academic Emergency Medicine (SAEM). Available at: http://www.saem.org/e-advising-faqs-students. Accessed February 9, 2012.

[59]American College of Physicians. Finding the right mentor for you. Available at: http://www.acponline.org/medical_students/impact/archives/2010/11/feature/. Accessed February 9, 2012.

[60]Association of Women Surgeons. Available at: https://www.womensurgeons.org/CDR/Mentorship.asp. Accessed February 9, 2012.

[61]Fahrenkopf A, Sectish T, Barger L, Sharek P, Lewin D, Chiang V, Edwards S, Wiedermann B, Landrigan C. Rates of medication errors among depressed and burnt out residents: prospective cohort study. *BMJ* 2008; 336(7642): 488-91.

[62]Wolf T, Faucett J, Randall H, Balson P. Graduating medical students' ratings of stresses, pleasures, and coping strategies. *J Med Educ* 1988; 63(8): 636-42.

[63]Compton M, Carrera J, Frank E. Stress and depressive symptoms/dysphoria among US medical students: results from a large, nationally representative survey. *J Nerv Ment Dis* 2008; 196(12): 891-7.

[64]Dyrbye L, Thomas M, Huntington J, Lawson K, Novotny P, Sloan J, Shanafelt T. Personal life events and medical student burnout: a multicenter study. *Acad Med* 2006; 81 (4): 374-84.

[65]Hussein E, Gabr A, Mohamed A, Hameed A. Physical exercise and anxiety among medical students at Ain Shams University. Presented at the 13th Annual International Ain Shams Medical Students' Congress, Feb 14-16, 2005.

[66]Parkerson G, Broadhead W, Tse C. The health status and life satisfaction of first-year medical students. *Acad Med* 1990; 65(9): 586-8.

[67]Carver C. You want to measure coping but your protocol's too long: consider the brief COPE. *International Journal of Behavioral Medicine* 1997; 4: 92-100.

[68]Gentile J, Roman B. Medical student mental health services; psychiatrists treating medical students. *Psychiatry* 2009; 6(5): 38-45.

[69]Baernstein A, Oelschlager A, Chang T, Wenrich M. Learning professionalism: perspectives of preclinical medical students. *Acad Med* 2009; 84(5): 574-81.

[70]Satterwhite W, Satterwhite R, Enarson C. Medical students' perceptions of unethical conduct at one medical school. *Acad Med* 1998; 73(5): 529-531.

[71]Humphrey H, Smith K, Reddy S, Scott D, Madara J, Arora V. Promoting an environment of professionalism: The University of Chicago "Roadmap." *Acad Med* 2007; 82(11): 1098-1107.

[72]Dans P. Self-reported cheating by students at one medical school. *Acad Med* 1996; 71 (1, suppl): S70-72.

[73]Anderson R, Obenshain S. Cheating by students: findings, reflections, and remedies. *Acad Med* 1994; 69(5): 323-332.

[74]Szauter K, Turner H. Using students' perceptions of internal medicine teachers' professionalism. *Acad Med* 2001; 76(5): 575-6.

[75]Kowalczyk L. Doctor accused of faking studies. *The Boston Globe*; March 11, 2009.

[76]Lin S, Strom S, Canales C, Rodriguez A, Kain Z. The impact of the anesthesiology clerkship structure on medical students matched to anesthesiology. Abstract presented at the 2010 Annual Meeting of the American Society Anesthesiologists. A1106.

[77]Kassebaum D, Szenas P. Medical students' career indecision and specialty rejection: roads not taken. *Acad Med* 1995; 70(10): 937-43.

[78]Association of American Medical Colleges. Available at: http://www.aamc.org/students/cim/august10choices.pdf. Accessed November 21, 2011.

[79]Association of American Medical Colleges (AAMC). Available at: http://www.aamc.org/students/cim/about.htm. Accessed September 23, 2011.

[80]University of Virginia School of Medicine Medical Specialty Aptitude Test. Available at: http://www.med-ed.virginia.edu/specialties. Accessed January 24, 2012.

[81]2010 AAMC Medical School Graduation Questionnaire. Available at: http://www.aamc.org. Accessed August 13, 2011.

[82]Dorsay E, Jarjoura D, Rutecki G. Influence of controllable lifestyle on recent trends in specialty choice by US medical students. *JAMA* 2003; 290(9): 1173-8.

[83]Weinstein P, Gipple C. Some determinants of career choice in the second year of medical school. *J Med Educ* 1975; 50(2): 194-8.

[84]Garmel G. Mentoring medical students in academic emergency medicine. *Acad Emerg Med* 2004; 11(12): 1351-7.

[85]ACP Mentoring Database. Available at: http://www.acponline.org/residents+fellows/mentors/. Accessed January 25, 2012.

An excerpt from the best-selling book:
Medical School Scholarships, Grants, &
Awards*:*
*Insider Advice on How to Win
Scholarships*

By Dr. Samir P. Desai

Medical School Scholarships & Awards

Note: The following chapter is excerpted from the book – Medical School Scholarships, Grants, & Awards: Insider Advice on How to Win Scholarships

According to the Association of American Medical Colleges (AAMC), the median four-year cost to attend medical school for the class of 2014 was over $218,000 and $286,000 for public and private schools, respectively.[1] The following table shows how the median cost of attendance has changed over time.

Change in 4-Year Median Cost to Attend Medical School (AAMC Data)[1-2]		
Year	Public	Private
2000	$100,215	$161,760
2008	$159,396	$225,215
2014	$218,898	$286,806

Although the average annual cost to attend medical school has risen at a rate that has outpaced inflation, this has not prevented a record number of students from applying to medical school. In 2013, there were over 48,000 applicants to U.S. medical schools, breaking the mark set in 1996.

Medical schools have been graduating more students than ever, the result of a nationwide effort to meet the needs of an anticipated physician manpower shortage. As these students fulfill their professional dreams of becoming physicians, they leave medical school with considerable debt. AAMC research indicates that the median education debt for the class of 2013 was $175,000.[1]

Fortunately, there are hundreds of scholarships available to medical students to help offset the cost of medical school education. Although there are few "full-ride" scholarships, there are many awards that can significantly lessen the burden. "Every $1,000 in scholarship support reduces a student's potential indebtedness by more than $8,400," writes the Wake Forest School of Medicine.[3]

Although financial relief is a major reason to pursue scholarships, the benefits of receiving such awards and honors extend well beyond money. Does winning a medical student award or scholarship make a difference in the residency match? It certainly does with multiple research studies demonstrating that awards provide a competitive edge.

        Election to the Alpha Omega Alpha Honor Medical Society (AOA) is
perhaps the most well studied award as it relates to residency admission.
Eligibility is limited to only allopathic medical students, and members are
selected based on academic achievement, leadership, professionalism, and
commitment to service by school chapters. According to the AOA Constitution,
no more than 1/6 of the graduating class can be elected into the school's chapter.
In 2012, the National Resident Matching Program, the organization that
administers the Match, surveyed 1,960 residency programs representing 21
specialties about the importance of various residency selection criteria.[4] Overall,
membership in AOA was cited by 51% as a factor in selecting applicants to
interview. Membership in AOA was also an important factor in the ranking of
applicants. Overall, it received a mean rating of 3.4 on a scale of 1 (not at all
important) to 5 (very important). Data for the individual specialties is presented
in the table on the following page.

Percentage Of Residency Programs Citing AOA As A Factor In Selecting Applicants To Interview By Specialty[4]	
Specialty	% of Programs
Anesthesiology	69%
Dermatology	57%
Emergency Medicine	57%
Family Medicine	24%
General Surgery	60%
Internal Medicine	51%
Neurosurgery	76%
Obstetrics & Gynecology	47%
Orthopaedic Surgery	68%
Otolaryngology	76%
Pathology	40%
Pediatrics	55%
Physical Medicine & Rehabilitation	26%
Plastic Surgery	75%
Psychiatry	38%
Radiation Oncology	61%
Radiology	66%

Although osteopathic students are not eligible for AOA induction, both
allopathic and osteopathic students may be elected into the Gold Humanism
Honor Society (GHHS). Started in 2002 by the Arnold P. Gold Foundation,
GHHS honors medical students for "demonstrated excellence in clinical care,
leadership, compassion and dedication to service."[5] In a study conducted to
determine if GHHS membership influences residency selection, the authors
wrote that "membership in GHHS may set candidates apart from their peers and
allow PDs to distinguish objectively the candidates who demonstrate
compassionate medical care."[6] In the 2012 NRMP Program Director Survey,

23% reported using Gold Society Membership as a factor in selecting applicants to interview.[4]

AOA and GHHS are not the only awards or honors viewed favorably by residency programs. In a survey of over 1,200 residency program directors in 21 specialties, Dr. Marianne Green, Associate Dean of Medical Education at the Northwestern University Feinberg School of Medicine, determined the relative importance of various residency selection criteria.[7] Dr. Green found that medical school awards (non-AOA) were tenth in importance among a group of 14 residency selection criteria. Although not as important as USMLE Step 1 scores, clerkship grades, and letters of recommendation, awards were ranked higher than such factors as preclinical grades, research while in medical school, and published medical school research.

Benefits of winning medical school awards and scholarships include the following:

- Awards can provide a significant boost to the strength of your residency application, and distinguish you from your peers. Awards and scholarships can easily be placed in the residency application, MSPE (Dean's Letter), letters of recommendation, and CV. We have found that interviewers often ask about awards during residency interviews.

Did you know...

In 2013, Justin Berk, a medical student at Texas Tech University School of Medicine, received the American Medical Association Foundation National Leadership Award. "For Justin, it's obviously a huge accolade and something that will follow him for the rest of his medical career," said Dr. Tedd Mitchell, President of Texas Tech Health Sciences Center, in an interview with *The Daily Toreador*. "As he's applying for residency programs, it will stand out."[8]

Did you know...

Alexander Gallan, a medical student at the Boston University School of Medicine, was the recipient of the 2012 American Society of Clinical Pathology Academic Excellence Award. "The award was a common topic during my residency interviews. I believe it helped my residency application immeasurably by providing justification for all the hard work I have done."[9]

- Competitive specialties and residency programs value students who have been recognized with awards. There is belief among educators that you will make similar contributions as a trainee.

Did you know...

When Casey DeDeugd, a medical student at the University of Central Florida, won the Medical Student Achievement Award from the Ruth Jackson Orthopaedic Society, she enhanced her visibility in the field. "Your accomplishments thus far are very impressive!" wrote Dr. Gloria Gogola, Chair of the Society's Scientific Committee. "We look forward...to welcoming you to our field of orthopaedic surgery."[10]

Did you know...

In 2008, Brian Caldwell, a medical student at the University of Arkansas for Medical Sciences, was the winner of the Dr. Constantin Cope Medical Student Research Award from the Society of Interventional Radiology. "Brian carried the whole project with very little help and really did a nice job," said Dr. William Culp, Professor of Radiology and Surgery. "I am so pleased that he won the national SIR award, because his participation in the conference introduced him to national leaders in interventional radiology and will help jumpstart his career."[11]

- You gain visibility in your school, and bring recognition to the institution.

Did you know...

When Ramy El-Diwany, an M.D./Ph.D. student at Johns Hopkins University, won the 2014 Excellence in Public Health Award from the U.S. Public Health Service (USPHS) Physician Professional Advisory Committee, his institution was also lauded. "This award is a testament to the education provided by the Johns Hopkins University School of Medicine and to the high caliber of its students," wrote USPHS Lt. Cmdr. Kimberly Smith. "We hope that this award will encourage other Johns Hopkins faculty and students to continue their strong work in public health."[12]

Did you know...

After Rahul Vanjani received the AMA Foundation Leadership Award, Dr. Scott Schroth, Senior Associate Dean of Academic Affairs at George Washington University, took pride in his student's accomplishment. "Rahul's commitment to the community and leadership of service efforts are unparalleled. He exemplifies the sort of creativity and dedication that we look for in medical students at GW, and we are extraordinarily proud of him as a winner of the AMA Foundation's 2011 Leadership Award."[13]

- Recipients have found that awards have made them more attractive for other awards and scholarships. Awards follow you throughout your career, and can make you more competitive for future opportunities, programs, and employment.

- You further your professional reputation and enhance your credibility in the areas that form the basis for the award.

- Winning an award or scholarship can give you the confidence to pursue other goals.

- Applying for an award requires the support of advocates who become reference letter writers. Strengthening these relationships over time allows faculty members to write strong letters of recommendation for residency.

Did you know...

In applying for awards, you often have to submit reference letters. Over time, your letter writers become even stronger advocates with a vested interest in furthering your career. After David Leverenz won the Southwestern Medical Foundation Ho Din Award, his mentor had this to say. "Dr. Leverenz has done exceptionally well in medical school, performed research, worked, volunteered, and completed multiple mission trips," said Dr. David Balis, his faculty mentor at UT Southwestern Medical Center. "But what strikes me most about David is his caring, sincere, compassionate personality." Dr. Leverenz is now a resident at Vanderbilt University.[14]

Did you know...

Winning a scholarship may also affect the way in which you view your specialty choice. "This scholarship has allowed me the freedom to broaden my thoughts about what field I want to pursue," said Mike Bosworth, a medical student at Tulane University. "My focus is more on how I can help patients versus what I can make."[15]

It is clear that there are compelling reasons to pursue medical school scholarships, awards, and grants. In this book, we'll show you how to maximize your chances of winning these awards. Although our book includes an extensive list of scholarships and awards, we've also placed considerable emphasis on strategy. Some examples of what you'll find in our book include:

- Although we encourage you to apply for the most competitive scholarships and awards, we also show you how to identify awards that are easier to win. There is considerably less competition for these awards, and we'll show you how you can significantly enhance your chances of winning.

- Since letters of recommendation are a critical component of most scholarship applications, how can you work closely with your letter writers to have the best possible letters written?

- The personal essay is an opportunity for you to stand out from the rest of the applicant field. What's the best approach to take with the essay? What makes an essay particularly compelling to the scholarship committee? How can you avoid common errors?

- Scholarship programs may ask you to submit a CV or enter information from your CV directly into the application. Content and appearance are important factors in the way your CV will be assessed, and we'll show you how to create one with maximum impact.

Our recommendations are based on data from a full spectrum of sources. Whenever possible, we present evidence obtained from scientific study and published in the academic medical literature. We also take an insider's look at the entire process based on our experiences. For years, we've helped applicants match successfully into competitive specialties and residency programs. We've worked with medical students at all levels, and we always try to identify scholarship and award programs that will bolster their credentials. In the process of helping students win scholarships and awards, we've gained insight into the factors that lead to success. There's much that can be learned from your predecessors, and we've included the profiles of past scholarship winners. Reading about their stories will help guide your strategy and application. Although it's been a joy for us to help medical students win scholarships and awards, we know that the process is difficult. Although success is never guaranteed, our advice and perspectives provide the specific, concrete recommendations that will maximize your chances of being an award recipient.

A Medical Student Scholarship Winner Speaks...

"The scholarship will greatly ease the trouble and distraction of growing debt so that I can focus on my studies, my family and my community. It is a generous gift, and I am reminded that it is an investment in my future. I know that it is my role in the future to give back to my community as a physician."[16]

Chapter excerpted from the book – Medical School Scholarships, Grants, & Awards: Insider Advice on How to Win Scholarships

An excerpt from the best-selling book:
Success on the Wards:
250 Rules for Clerkship Success

By Dr. Samir P. Desai
and Dr. Rajani Katta

Introduction

Rule # 1   **You came to medical school to be a great doctor. That process begins now.**

Why did you become a doctor? There may be a number of reasons, but the most important one is the same across the board: to take care of patients. You will read startling amounts of information during medical school, and your training will include many procedures and new techniques, but all of it is in the service of patient care. You are here to make each and every individual patient better.

That process starts now.

It is an amazing privilege to take care of patients. You can read about a disease all that you want, but to be able to speak to and examine a patient with that disease is an unsurpassed learning experience. It is an incredible responsibility as well. You will be asking patients the most intimate and intrusive types of questions. You will be asking patients to offer their arm for a needle, to disrobe for an exam, to let you literally poke and prod at their body. In return, you are responsible for protecting them from harm, and for healing them.

Starting as a medical student, and progressing to a respected physician, is a long, difficult, and intense process. It takes years of education, and years of training. The privileges granted to physicians are remarkable. In return, you have a great responsibility. Your education is in the service of patient care. You have a responsibility to make the most of that education.

What does it take to be a great doctor? There is an impressive body of research devoted to medical student education, and to the factors and interventions that ensure good doctors. Medical educators work hard to ensure that students master these different facets of the practice of medicine.

Why are clerkships so important to the process of producing great doctors?

The areas emphasized in clerkships are those that are integral to becoming a great physician.

Patient care requires the daily use of many skills. On a daily basis, a physician may need to:

- Obtain an accurate medication history.
- Detect a heart murmur.
- Create a differential diagnosis for the patient with abdominal pain.
- Interpret an elevated alkaline phosphatase.
- Formulate a management plan for the patient with a myocardial infarction.
- Communicate that plan through oral discussions and written documentation.
- Utilize the talents of an entire health care team to maximize patient care.
- Manifest their concern for the patient in every interaction.

Clerkships teach students how to accomplish these difficult, vital skills.

If you don't learn certain skills in medical school, you may never learn them.

Clinical clerkships provide the foundation of successful patient care. They represent a critical time in your education. If you want to become proficient in exam skills, you have to learn now. These aren't skills you can learn from reading a textbook. You need to evaluate patients with these findings, and you need to have a teacher that can demonstrate these findings. You need to be able to ask questions freely in order to learn all the finer points of physical exam skills. This isn't something you can easily do as a resident, and certainly not as a board-certified physician. If you don't know how to assess jugular venous distention by the end of medical school, you may never learn.

While you would assume that medical school teaches you everything you need to know to function well as a resident, that isn't true for all students, particularly those who take a passive approach to learning or those who focus their education on textbook learning. You need to maximize your learning experiences and teaching opportunities on the wards. Passive learning has real consequences.

In one eye-opening study, internal medicine residents were tested on cardiac auscultatory skills. They listened to 12 prerecorded cardiac events. American residents demonstrated poor proficiency, with mean identification rates of only 22%.[1] In another study of resident skills, ECG proficiency was measured. Surprisingly, 58% of residents wrongly diagnosed complete heart block, and only 22% were certain of their diagnosis of ventricular tachycardia.[2] In a study of radiologic proficiency, participants included mainly residents, with some students. In x-rays representing emergency situations, pneumothorax was misdiagnosed by 91% of participants overall, while a misplaced central venous catheter was missed by 74%.[3]

Skills in patient examination, interpretation of tests, synthesis of information, and medical decision-making are honed through years of practice. Clerkships are only the first step, but provide an invaluable education, with supervisors there to demonstrate, to model, and to teach skills. The best medical students regard clerkships as a unique and invaluable learning experience, difficult to replicate in residency or later through seminars and conferences.

If you don't learn it now, you may have problems as a resident.

Medical school is the time to learn and develop your clinical skills. It's also the time to develop and hone the learned attributes and attitudes that predict success as a physician. In a study of residents with problematic behavior, investigators sought to determine if there were prognostic indicators in their medical school evaluations.[4] The short answer is yes.

Students whose evaluations indicated that they were timid, had problems in organization, displayed little curiosity, and had difficulty applying knowledge clinically, among other types, were more likely to become problem residents. The authors "found a rather robust multilevel correlation between residents who have problems, major or minor, during or after residency, and negative statements, even subtle ones, in the dean's letter." The predictive statements noted in the dean's letter included:

Very nervous, timid initially/ Displayed little curiosity/ Had difficulty applying knowledge clinically/ He came across as confrontational/ Maybe somewhat overconfident for his level of training/ Lack of enthusiasm and problems in organization/
Needs to read more on her own/ Lots of effort, uneven outcome

Difficulties during clerkships may predict difficulties as a physician, including disciplinary actions by the State Medical Board.

Clerkships are the foundation of successful patient care. During clerkships, medical students also develop and hone the attributes and attitudes that are required of successful physicians. These are referred to collectively as medical professionalism. "The specific attributes that have long been understood to animate professionalism include altruism, respect, honesty, integrity, dutifulness, honour, excellence and accountability."[5] –Dr. Jordan Cohen, President Emeritus, Association of American Medical Colleges

If you don't hone these traits during medical school, you may have problems as a physician. Unprofessional behavior in medical school is a possible predictor of future disciplinary action. A particularly notable study was performed by Dr. Maxine Papadakis, associate dean for student affairs at the UCSF School of Medicine. She and her team examined the medical school records of 235 graduates of three medical schools. Each of these physicians had been disciplined by one of 40 state medical boards over a 13-year period. The disciplined physicians were three times more likely than a control group to have negative comments about their professionalism documented in their medical school record.[6]

Another study sought to identify the domains of unprofessional behavior in medical school that were associated with disciplinary action by a state medical board.[7] Three domains of unprofessional behavior were significantly associated with future disciplinary action: poor reliability and responsibility, poor initiative and motivation, and lack of self-improvement and adaptability.

Your core clerkship grades may either limit or expand your future career options.

The skills and traits reflected in core clerkship grades are considered so important to future success as a resident that residency programs use these grades as a major criteria in the selection process. Program directors are decision-makers in the residency selection process. In a survey of over 1,200 residency program directors across 21 medical specialties, grades in required clerkships were ranked as the # 1 factor used in the selection process.[8]

Studies across multiple specialties have supported the predictive nature of clerkship grades. In one study, researchers sought to determine which residency selection criteria had the strongest correlation with performance as an orthopedic surgery resident. The authors concluded that the "number of honors grades on clinical rotations was the strongest predictor of performance."[9] In a study of physical medicine and rehabilitation residents, "clinical residency performance was predicted by clerkship grade honors."[10] In one study of internal medicine residents, performance as a resident was significantly associated with the internal medicine clerkship grade.[11]

In the next 400 plus pages, we review each of the areas that students need to master in clerkships. The book contains a great deal of in-depth content across a range of areas vital to medical student success. It's also arranged to ensure ease of use. The first sections serve as straightforward how-to guides for each of the core clerkships. If you're starting your Pediatrics clerkship, and aren't sure how to write the daily patient progress note, Chapter 4 walks you through that process. If you're starting the Ob/Gyn clerkship, and don't know how to write a delivery note, Chapter 6 provides a template and sample note that details exactly what you'll need to include. The latter chapters provide more wide-ranging content. If you'll be presenting in rounds for the first time, you can turn to the chapter on oral case presentations and review the features you'll need to include. If you are committed to fully protecting your patients from the hazards of hospitalization, Chapter 8 Patients includes several tables that outline the steps that medical students can take, even at their level, to protect their patients. Chapter 22 reviews the impact of collaborative care on patient outcomes, and provides recommendations that students can implement.

The recommendations presented here are based on discussions with numerous faculty members, residents, and students, as well as our own experiences. We've also focused our efforts on evidence-based advice. This evidence-based advice is based on our review of the substantial medical literature in the area of medical student education. The book includes over 400 references from the relevant literature.

Over the next 400 plus pages, you'll learn how to maximize your education during core clerkships, as well as your performance. Your success on the wards will become the foundation of outstanding patient care.

Patients

We begin this chapter with one of the most famous quotes in the history of medicine. "First, do no harm." From ancient times onwards, medical practice has posed dangers to patients. In modern times, those dangers are shockingly common. Medical error is thought to be the third leading case of death in the US.[12] Those errors include the unbelievable: one report described an average of 27 cases in one year, per New York hospital, of invasive procedures performed on the wrong patient.[13] Some of those dangers have become so commonplace that we consider them routine. When a patient develops a hospital-related infection, we document it as a nosocomial infection and treat the infection without questioning why it occurred. However, many of those infections are preventable, and should never have occurred at all. In this chapter, we document a number of specific measures that medical students can implement to protect their patients, from the use of standardized abbreviations to ensuring that patients receive venous thromboembolism prophylaxis when indicated. We outline how medical students can identify the hazards of hospitalization, thus ensuring that you can act to mitigate those hazards. We review nosocomial infections, and how you may be a culprit through your hands, your clothing, and even your stethoscope.

We also review the type of skills that ensure that patients feel comfortable with your care. The best medical care necessitates that patients trust their physicians and have confidence in both their abilities and the fact that the physician cares about the patient, not just the illness. In this chapter, our focus is on the patient, and how medical students can improve the care provided to patients. We outline steps that students can take, even at their level, to protect their patients from physical harm. We emphasize the different ways in which medical students can enhance patient care, patient education, and patient counseling. On a daily basis, you have the opportunity and the power to enhance the care provided to your patients.

Internal Medicine Clerkship

The field of internal medicine (IM) has a broad impact on all fields of medicine. "Learning about internal medicine – the specialty providing comprehensive care to adults – in the third year of medical school is an important experience, regardless of what specialty the medical student ultimately pursues," says Dr. Patrick Alguire, the Director of Education and Career Development at the American College of Physicians.[14] Through this clerkship, you will hone your skills in history and physical examination, diagnostic test interpretation, medical decision-making, and management of core medical conditions. These skills are important ones for all physicians, even if you ultimately decide to enter radiology, pathology, emergency medicine, or another field. Overall, internal medicine does stand as the most frequently chosen specialty in the residency match. In 2010, over 3,000 allopathic and osteopathic medical students matched into an internal medicine residency program.

Your IM clerkship grade can impact your career. It's a factor in the residency selection process for all specialties, not just internal medicine. In a survey of over 1,200 residency program directors across 21 medical specialties, grades in required clerkships were ranked as the

1 factor used in the selection process.[8] "Do well in your clerkship," writes the Department of Medicine at the University of Washington. "Yes, this is obvious – and easier said than done – but it's also important. Most residency programs look closely at the third-year clerkship grade when selecting applicants."[15]

Many medical students find this clerkship formidable. A lack of knowledge isn't the main factor. The main factor is a lack of preparation for your many responsibilities. How do I evaluate a newly admitted patient? What do I need to include in a daily progress note? What information do I need to include in a comprehensive write-up? How do I present newly admitted patients to the attending physician?

In this chapter, templates and outlines are included for each of these important responsibilities. You'll also find a number of tips and suggestions on how to maximize your learning and performance during this rotation. You'll find detailed information that will help you effectively pre-round, succeed during work rounds, deliver polished oral case presentations, create well-written daily progress notes, and generate comprehensive write-ups.

For students interested in a career in internal medicine, this chapter also details how to strengthen your application. You'll learn how to identify potential mentors and obtain strong letters of recommendation. You'll learn about recommended electives and sub-internships, as well as specifics that detail how to maximize the impact of your application.

Surgery Clerkship

The surgery clerkship provides significant exposure to common surgical problems, and allows you to evaluate the specialty as a potential career choice. Although the bulk of your education will take place on the general surgery service, most rotations provide the opportunity to explore several surgical subspecialties. A surgical clerkship education is very valuable, whether or not you choose to practice in a surgical field. Primary care physicians must be familiar with the evaluation and management of patients in the pre-operative and post-operative settings. An understanding of core surgical principles is important across many fields, including ones such as anesthesiology, dermatology, and emergency medicine. From a personal standpoint, you or a family member is likely to undergo surgery in your lifetime, and you'll find that an understanding of the pre-operative, operative, and post-operative stages will be valuable.

Regardless of your chosen career, your surgery clerkship grade will be a factor used in the residency selection process, due to an emphasis on core clerkship grades in the residency selection process. In a survey of over 1,200 residency program directors across 21 medical specialties, grades in required clerkships were ranked as the # 1 factor used in the selection process.[8] The University of Colorado Department of Surgery writes that "most surgery programs look very favorably on an 'Honors' grade in your MS3 surgery clerkship rotation and may factor in the grades you received in your Medicine and Ob/Gyn rotations."[16] It's not easy to honor the clerkship. In a survey of medical schools across the country, Takayama found that only 27% of students achieve the highest grade in the surgery clerkship.[17]

Many students approach the surgery clerkship with considerable anxiety. In one study, students were most concerned about fatigue, long hours, workload, insufficient sleep, lack of time to study, mental abuse (getting yelled at or relentless pimping), and poor performance.[18] Unfamiliarity with the operating room environment was also concerning.

In the Surgery Clerkship chapter, we provide tips for operating room success, a checklist for thorough pre-rounding, a step-by-step guide to presenting patients, and time-saving templates for the pre-op, post-op, and op notes. This information will maximize your education as well as your performance.

In 2010, approximately 2,500 allopathic and osteopathic medical students matched into general surgery or related surgical specialty, such as ophthalmology, orthopedic surgery, otolaryngology, plastic surgery, or urology. This chapter includes recommendations for those students interested in pursuing general surgery as a career. When should you do a sub-internship? Should you do an away elective? What are considered negatives in a residency application? These questions, and others, are answered.

Excerpted from the book *Success on the Wards: 250 Rules for Clerkship Success.*

An excerpt from the best-selling book:
The Successful Match 2017:
Rules for Success in the Residency Match

By Dr. Rajani Katta
and Dr. Samir P. Desai

Introduction

What does it take to match successfully? What does it take to match into the specialty and program of your choice?

Over 42,000 applicants registered for the 2016 NRMP Match, making it the largest Match on record. Competition is intense, and some applicants are unsuccessful.[1]

In competitive fields such as general surgery, dermatology, plastic surgery, and orthopedic surgery, over 25% of U.S. senior allopathic applicants failed to match.

Overall, while nearly 94% of U.S. allopathic senior applicants matched, the number of unmatched seniors reached an all-time high of 1,130 applicants. The numbers are significantly worse for osteopathic and international medical graduates (IMGs). Failure to match rates are shown in the following tables.

Percentage of U.S. Allopathic Senior Applicants Who Failed to Match in Competitive Specialties (2016 NRMP and AUA Match)[2-3]	
Specialty	**% of U.S. Seniors Failing to Match**
Dermatology	28%
General Surgery	27%
Orthopedic Surgery	26%
Plastic Surgery	25%
Neurological Surgery	25%
Urology	23%
Radiation Oncology	19%
Otolaryngology	13%

Failure to Match % by Applicant Type (2016 NRMP Match)[2]	
Applicant Type	**% Failing to Match**
Osteopathic applicants	20%
U.S. citizen IMGs	46%
Non-U.S. citizen IMGs	50%

Did you know?

The failure to match rates reported by the NRMP for competitive specialties don't take into account the following:

- Applicants who give up on their preferred specialty choice because they feel that their chances of success are low.
- Applicants who apply to their preferred specialty choice but fail to receive an interview.

These applicants don't officially enter the match for their preferred specialty, and are therefore not included in these statistics. Some researchers have therefore looked at "intent to match" failure rates, and those rates are indeed significantly higher.

As an applicant, your goal is to match into your preferred specialty, and ideally your preferred program.

The evidence indicates that it has never been more difficult to reach these goals.

Over a decade ago, in response to an anticipated physician manpower shortage, allopathic and osteopathic medical schools increased student enrollment. New schools were also established. However, the number of residency positions has not increased at a corresponding rate. As more and more graduates have entered the Match, the competition for available residency positions has intensified.

Did you know?

In a 2015 survey of medical school deans, the AAMC asked "What is your level of concern about your incoming students' ability to find a residency training position of their choice upon completion of medical school?" 50% of the deans surveyed indicated having "major" or "moderate" concern. Of note, the percentage reporting this degree of concern rose from 35% in 2012 to 50% in 2015.[4]

What does it take to match successfully in such a fiercely competitive environment?

The issue is a hotly debated one, and surveys of students, reviews of student discussion forums, and discussions with academic faculty all find sharp divisions on the topic. Try entering this subject into a search engine, and you'll receive thousands of conflicting opinions.

I was speaking to a colleague, and I brought up this question and my work on this book. Her response? "A book on matching? What's there to write about? Get good grades and a great score on the USMLE. That's the book!"

Her response was sadly misinformed.

There's no doubt that medical school grades and USMLE Step 1 scores are very important, but focusing only on those two factors certainly doesn't tell the full story. If that were the case, it wouldn't explain these cases:

- A student with a Step 1 score of 260, membership in AOA, and published dermatology research, was only invited to interview at 2 dermatology programs (one of which was his home school).

- Another student, with a Step 1 score of 230 and no AOA membership, was invited to 9 dermatology interviews.

- Another student with great scores – but minimal dermatology research – was invited to interview at over 20 dermatology programs.

From a scientific approach, what are the factors that account for so much of the variability in match outcomes?

That's an interesting question, but I'm very interested in this topic for a far more personal reason. How can I help this student, sitting across my desk, match into dermatology? This is a very important, personal question for me.

After 17 years as a faculty member, and at a school that fields a high number of dermatology applicants (some years we've had as many as 12 applicants), I've advised many applicants. Dr. Samir Desai has advised a wide cross-section of applicants, from applicants with 15 interview invitations to those reapplying for the 4th time. Together, we've advised hundreds of applicants.

I certainly don't think you need an incredible USMLE score to be a great dermatologist, and yet that's being used as a screen by so many programs. I think we're missing some great applicants because of it. My goal is to help those applicants who I think will make great contributions to the care of their patients and to the specialty: conscientious, thorough, empathetic, and with a strong sense of intellectual curiosity. How can I, as an advisor, help such students? How can you, as that type of student, reach your professional goals?

The first edition of this book was published in 2009, and while the core strategies for a successful match remain the same, some important changes have occurred. The most relevant is that the competition is more intense.

With increased competition, it has become even more important to ensure that your application stands out from the other 499 applications that your dream program has received.

What does it take to achieve a successful match? It takes the right strategy. It also takes significant advanced planning and hard work, above and beyond the intense coursework of medical school.

In the following 600 plus pages, we answer the question of what it takes to match successfully. We also provide specific evidence-based advice to maximize your chances of a successful match.

Our recommendations are based on data from a full spectrum of sources. We present evidence obtained from scientific study and published in the academic medical literature. The results of these studies can provide a powerful impetus for specific actions. We present anecdotal data and advice that have been published in the literature and obtained from online sources. We also take an insider's look at the entire process of residency selection based on our experiences, the experiences of our colleagues in the world of academic medicine, and the experiences of the students and residents with whom we've worked.

We focus on the important questions that define the optimal match strategy. Who are the decision-makers? What criteria do they value? How can you ensure that your application materials highlight these criteria?

Who actually chooses the residents? We review the data on the decision-makers. What do these decision-makers care about? We review the data on the criteria that matter to them. How can you convince them that you would be the right resident for their program? We provide concrete, practical recommendations based on this data. At every step of the process, our recommendations are meant to maximize the impact of your application.

In Chapters 23 - 44, we present specialty-specific data. Given the high failure to match rates for certain specialties, is there any literature available to applicants to guide them through the residency application process? For each specialty, we present the results of those studies. For example, in urology, a survey of residency program directors (PDs) obtained data from 76 directors on the criteria that programs use to select their residents.[5] What criteria did these directors rank as most important in deciding whom to interview? Which selection factors were most important in determining an applicant's place on the program's rank order list? What were the factors that led programs to downgrade applicants? This evidence-based information is critical to developing an application strategy that maximizes your chances of a successful match.

We review each component of the application in comprehensive detail in the following chapters. Each and every component of your application can be created, modified, or influenced in order to significantly enhance your overall candidacy. We devote the next 600 plus pages of this book to showing you, in detail, exactly how to do so.

Overview of Book

The first edition of this book was written in 2009, and we've seen a sharp rise in the competitiveness of many specialties since that time. This has translated to applicants applying more widely and extensively than ever before. This means that programs are receiving a record number of applications, and it's become ever more difficult to stand out in this sea of applications.

Increasing Competition for Residency Positions	
Residency Program	**Comments**
Department of Anesthesiology Ohio State University	"Anesthesiology is not the most competitive field, but it has become a lot more competitive in recent years."[6]
Department of EM UCSF	"Emergency Medicine residency programs are becoming increasingly more competitive. This field is more popular than in the past, leading to a robust number of applicants each year. There are generally very few positions to 'scramble' into each year."[7]
Department of Surgery University of Colorado	"Over the past five years, general surgery has become quite competitive."[8]

Did you know?

In the 2016 Match, 47% of all U.S. allopathic senior applicants failed to match at the program of their choice.[2]

This has led applicants to submit a larger number of applications to programs, as shown in the following table.

Average Number of Applications Per Applicant (2011 Versus 2015)[9]		
Specialty	**Average Number of Applications Per Applicant (2011)**	**Average Number of Applications Per Applicant (2015)**
Dermatology	40	60
Emergency Medicine	27	35
Obstetrics & Gynecology	32	40
Orthopedic Surgery	47	67
Otolaryngology	38	46
Radiation Oncology	28	35
Urology	44	58

The larger number of applications means more challenges for programs. Programs are finding it difficult to reduce this large group of applicants into a smaller, more manageable number who will receive interview invitations. "These additional applications…cause congestion in the application review process," writes Dr. Steven Weissbart. "Therefore program directors may overlook preferred applicants as a result."[10]

Did you know?

"As medical schools have increased their class sizes to address the demand for physicians and the number of residency slots has largely remained the same, students are forced to navigate the application process more strategically to match into residency programs."[11]

G. Scott Waterman, M.D.
Former Associate Dean for Student Affairs
University of Vermont

Personal Statement

For many students the most dreaded aspect of the residency application is the personal statement. If the words "personal statement" raise your anxiety level, you are certainly not alone. In a study of students at a single medical school, 85% agreed or strongly agreed with the following statement:[12]

I am anxious about writing the personal statement for my residency application.

Individual specialties, residency programs, and application reviewers assign varying degrees of importance to the personal statement. In the screening phase, reviewers whittle down a large applicant pool to a select group that is ultimately extended interview invitations. At some programs, the personal statement is used minimally, if at all, during this screening phase. In others, the personal statement is considered very important:

- "Program directors read a lot of personal statements, so make yours stand out," writes Dr. Jennifer Oman, former program director of the UC Irvine Emergency Medicine Residency Program. "This is something that you want to pour your heart into and give your full attention…Take the time to do this right. It can save a borderline application from being thrown into the rejection pile."[13]

- "The personal statement helps us to get to know you, and we read it with great care," writes Dr. Dempsey Springfield, Program Director of the Harvard Combined Orthopedics Program.[14]

- "This is your only chance to 'talk' to us – make the most of it…a really good statement could be just enough to tip the balance in your favor and move you into the interview pool," writes the Wake Forest University Department of Orthopedic Surgery.[15]

- The website for the University of Washington Family Medicine Residency states that the "personal statement is the primary component that will be used to select applicants who are invited for an interview. Please write a careful and thoughtful document."[16]

Adding to the importance of the personal statement is this fact: a poorly conceived and executed personal statement may be detrimental to your application. Otherwise excellent candidates have been ranked lower, or even rejected, because of a poorly written statement. As reinforced by the University of Alabama at Birmingham Department of Obstetrics and Gynecology – "poorly written personal statements may detract from an otherwise excellent application."[17] Even when statements are free of glaring errors, far too many are viewed as neutral, and this represents a lost opportunity to impress the program.

Applicants are urged by advisors and PDs to create thoughtful and unique statements. Crafting a compelling personal statement requires reflection and creative writing. The evidence indicates that many students are uncomfortable doing just that. In the aforementioned survey, only 29% agreed or strongly agreed with the following statement:[12]

I am comfortable with creative and reflective writing.

It is very frustrating trying to put into words your vision for your medical career. Most students don't understand one basic fact about the personal statement, though. Unlike just about every other aspect of the application, you have complete control over the personal statement. You decide the content, the structure, and the form of the statement. This is a unique opportunity to impress the selection committee. In your statement you can showcase your strengths and those qualities that set you apart from other candidates. You can weave in evidence that confirms your qualities. You can use this opportunity to convince a faculty member that you would be an ideal candidate for their particular program. This is information that is not readily apparent to programs from their review of other application components.

When you create a personal statement, you need to consider your audience. When reading a personal statement, what do faculty members look for? What are they trying to determine? Consider the following:

- In a study evaluating the content of personal statements, members of the radiology residency selection committee at Wayne State University ranked eleven content areas from least to most important.[18] Most important was a candidate's explanation as to why they chose to pursue a career in radiology. Personal attributes was second in importance, while perception of radiology defined as the applicant's ability "to explicitly state what he/she feels are the most important characteristics of either radiologists or the practice of radiology" was third.

- In a survey of orthopedic surgery PDs, 43% agreed that "the most important aspect of a personal statement is to learn more about the candidate's personal interests and backgrounds," while 32% stated that "the most important aspect of a personal statement was to gain insight into an applicant's ability to write and to communicate effectively."[19]

- Among 47 themes identified in an analysis of dermatology personal statements, three were found to be emphasized more often by applicants who matched (studying cutaneous manifestations of systemic disease, contributing to the literature gap, and investigating the pathophysiology of skin diseases).[20]

- At the website for the Wayne State University pathology residency, the program writes that "your personal statement should summarize your particular background and interests and depict you as a person. You should indicate in your personal statement why you are interested in Pathology, what kind of experience you have had with Pathology, and what career path you plan to follow after training."[21]

In our chapter on the personal statement (Chapter 7), we review in more detail what programs seek in the personal statement. We review different approaches and provide a springboard to brainstorming and developing your own statement. We review in detail how to conceive and execute a personal statement that reflects your individual strengths and skills, while convincingly conveying your excellent fit with the specialty and with the individual programs in a convincing manner.

Letters of Recommendation

Letters of recommendation (LORs) are a critical component of the residency application. In the 2014 NRMP Program Director Survey, 86% of programs in 22 specialties cited LORs as a factor in selecting applicants to interview.[22] The only factor cited more frequently by PDs was the USMLE Step 1 / COMLEX Level 1 score.

Since you won't be directly writing these letters yourself, it may seem as if you have no control over their content. In reality, you wield more influence than you realize. In our chapter on letters of recommendation, we detail the steps that you can take in order to have the best possible letters written on your behalf. These steps include choosing the correct letter writers and asking in the correct manner. We also discuss the type of information to provide, and the manner in which to provide it, in order to highlight those qualities that you hope your letter writer will emphasize.

The purpose of these letters is to emphasize that you have the professional qualifications needed to excel. The letters should also demonstrate that you have the personal qualities to succeed as a resident and, later, as a practicing physician. Since these letters are written by those who know you and the quality of your work, they offer programs a personalized view. In contrast to your transcript and USMLE scores, they supply programs with qualitative, rather than quantitative, information about your cognitive and non-cognitive characteristics.

What do the faculty members reviewing applications look for in a letter of recommendation? The first item noted is the writer of the letter. In a survey of PDs in four specialties (internal medicine, pediatrics, family medicine, and surgery), it was learned that a candidate's likelihood of being considered was enhanced if there was a connection or relationship between the writer and residency program director. "In cases where there was both a connection between the faculty members and in-depth knowledge of the student (i.e., personal

Excerpted from the book *The Successful Match 2017: Rules for Success in the Residency Match*.

Read more of the first chapter at www.TheSuccessfulMatch.com.

Medical School Interview: Winning Strategies from Admissions Faculty

By Samir Desai and Rajani Katta

ISBN # 9781937978013

The medical school interview is the most important factor in the admissions process. Our detailed advice, based on evidence from research in the field and the perspectives of admissions faculty, will provide you with the insiders' perspective.

How can you best prepare for the traditional interview, group interview, panel interview, and behavioral interview? What qualities would make applicants less likely to be admitted? What personal qualities are most valued by admissions faculty? What can students do to achieve maximum success during the interview?

This book shows medical school applicants how to develop the optimal strategy for interview success.

"…this is an extremely thorough handbook, covering the questions applicants are likely to be asked and the appropriate and inappropriate answers…likely to be found indispensable by readers embarking on the arduous process of applying to medical school."

-   Kirkus Reviews

Success in Medical School: Insider Advice for the Preclinical Years

By Samir P. Desai and Rajani Katta

ISBN # 9781937978006

According to the AAMC, the United States will have a shortage of 90,000 physicians by 2020. In the mid-1990s, the AAMC urged medical schools to expand enrollment. Class sizes have increased, and new schools have opened their doors. Unfortunately, rising enrollment in medical schools has not led to a corresponding increase in the number of residency positions.

As a result, medical students are finding it increasingly difficult to match with the specialty and program of their choice. "Competition is tightening," said Mona Signer, Executive Director of the National Resident Matching Program. "The growth in applicants is more than the increase in positions."

Now more than ever, preclinical students need to be well informed so that they can maximize their chances of success. The decisions you make early in medical school can have a significant impact on your future specialty options.

To build a strong foundation for your future physician career, and to match into your chosen field, you must maximize your preclinical education. In *Success in Medical School*, you'll learn specific strategies for success during these important years of medical school.

"Overall, I recommend this book...The book has so much information about everything that there has to be a part of the book that will satisfy your interests."

- Medical School Success website

Medical School Scholarships, Grants & Awards: Insider Advice On How To Win Scholarships

By Samir P. Desai and Anand Trivedi

ISBN # 9781937978044

Residency match expert Dr. Samir Desai has helped students win medical school scholarships, grants, and awards, and now shares his perspectives in this new resource.

Over 1,000 awards are featured along with profiles of winners, proven strategies for success, and crucial tips. Learn how to craft a powerful scholarship application, write compelling essays, secure strong letters of recommendation, and stand out from the competition. Discover the best scholarships for you with awards for research, leadership, writing, global health, service, extracurricular activities, ethnicity, and gender.

Winning can:

- Significantly reduce your debt.
- Provide a major boost to your residency application, and set you apart from your peers. Awards can be placed in the application, MSPE, letters of recommendation, and CV.
- Elevate your profile with competitive specialties and residency programs.
- Raise your stature in medical school.
- Make you more attractive for other awards and scholarships.
- Further your professional reputation and enhance your credibility in the areas that form the basis for the award.
- Solidify the support of faculty who become reference letter writers. Strengthening these relationships over time allows faculty members to write strong letters of recommendation for residency.

Clinician's Guide to Laboratory Medicine: Pocket

By Samir P. Desai

ISBN # 9780972556187

In this book, you will find practical approaches to lab test interpretation. It includes differential diagnoses, step-by-step approaches, and algorithms, all designed to answer your lab test questions in a flash. See why so many consider it a "must-have" book.

"In our Medicine Clerkship, the Clinician's Guide to Laboratory Medicine has quickly become one of the two most popular paperback books. Our students have praised the algorithms, tables, and ease of pursuit of clinical problems through better understanding of the utilization of tests appropriate to the problem at hand."

- Greg Magarian, MD, Director, 3rd Year Internal Medicine Clerkship, Oregon Health & Science University

"It provides an excellent practical approach to abnormal labs."

- Northwestern University Feinberg School of Medicine Internal Medicine Clerkship website.

Success on the Wards: 250 Rules for Clerkship Success

By Samir P. Desai and Rajani Katta

ISBN # 9780972556194

This is an absolute must-read for students entering clinical rotations.

The authors of *The Successful Match: 200 Rules to Succeed in the Residency Match* bring their same combination of practical recommendations and evidence-based advice to clerkships.

The book begins as a how-to guide with clerkship-specific templates, along with sample notes and guides, for every aspect of clerkships. The book reviews proven strategies for success in patient care, write-ups, rounds, and other vital areas.

Grades in required rotations are the most important academic criteria used to select residents, and this critical year can determine career choices. This book shows students what they can do now to position themselves for match success. An invaluable resource for medical students - no student should be without it.

"*Success on the Wards: 250 Rules for Clerkship Success* is an excellent reference for any 3rd year medical student and some is probably great reading for advanced students and even residents and interns…Given the heavy importance of being successful on the wards as a student for future residency, it's really easy to recommend this book."

-   Review by Medfools.com

"*Success on the Wards* is easily the best book I have read on how to succeed in clerkship. It is comprehensive, thorough and jam-packed with valuable information. Dr. Desai and Dr. Katta provide an all encompassing look into what clerkship is really like."

-   Review by Medaholic.com

The Successful Match 2017: Rules for Success in the Residency Match

By Rajani Katta and Samir P. Desai

ISBN # 9781937978075

What does it take to match into the specialty and program of your choice?

The key to a successful match hinges on the development of the right strategy. This book will show you how to develop the optimal strategy for success.

Who actually chooses the residents? We review the data on the decision-makers. What do these decision-makers care about? We review the data on the criteria that matter most to them. How can you convince them that you would be the right resident for their program? We provide concrete, practical recommendations based on their criteria.

At every step of the process, our recommendations are meant to maximize the impact of your application. This book is an invaluable resource to help you gain that extra edge.

"Drs. Rajani Katta and Samir P. Desai provide the medical student reader with detailed preparation for the matching process. The rules and accompanying tips make the book user-friendly. The format is especially appealing to those pressed for time or looking for a single key element for a particular process."

- Review in the American Medical Student Association journal, *The New Physician*

The Resident's Guide to the Fellowship Match

By Samir P. Desai

ISBN # 9781937978020

What does it take to match into the subspecialty and fellowship program of your choice?

Our detailed advice, based on evidence from research in the field and the perspectives of fellowship program directors, will provide you with the insiders' perspective.

What are criteria most important to decision-makers? What can you do to have the best possible letters of recommendation written on your behalf? How can you develop a powerful and compelling personal statement? How can you overcome the obstacles of residency to publish research? What can you do to achieve maximum success during the interview?

This book shows fellowship applicants how to develop the optimal strategy for success - an invaluable resource to help applicants gain that extra edge.

"The Resident's Guide to The Fellowship Match is a great book…It helps you prepare for the fellowship application starting on the first day of residency. I personally learned a lot from it…The book is very systematic and covers everything you need to ace your fellowship interviews. I would strongly recommend this book…"

- Huda Khaleel (Amazon Review)

The Successful Match website

Our website, TheSuccessfulMatch.com, provides medical school applicants with a better understanding of the admissions and selection process. You'll find:

- Inside look at the medical school admissions process
- Advice from the decision-makers
- Tips to help you tailor your interview answers from school to school
- Resources to help you succeed in the preclinical years and clerkships
- Information to position yourself for residency match success

Consulting services

We also offer expert one-on-one consulting services to premedical or medical students. For premedical students, editing services for the AMCAS application and personal statement are available. Dr. Desai and Dr. Katta also offer mock interview services based on years of experience interviewing applicants. They will offer you a detailed strategy for success tailored to your medical school of interest. We have the knowledge, expertise, and insight to help you achieve your goals. If you are interested in our consultation services, please visit us at www.TheSuccessfulMatch.com. The website provides further details, including pricing and specific services.

MD2B Titles

The Medical School Interview: Winning Strategies from Admissions Faculty

Medical School Scholarships, Grants, & Awards: Insider Advice on How to Win Scholarships

Success in Medical School: Insider Advice for the Preclinical Years

Success on the Wards: 250 Rules for Clerkship Success

The Successful Match 2017: Rules for Success in the Residency Match

Resident's Guide to the Fellowship Match: Rules for Success

Clinician's Guide to Laboratory Medicine: Pocket

Available at www.TheSuccessfulMatch.com

Bulk Sales

MD2B is able to provide discounts on any of our titles when purchased in bulk. The discount rate depends on the quantity ordered. For more information, please contact us at info@md2b.net or (713) 927-6830.